AF879943

PHYSEO

TABLE OF CONTENTS

We would like to extend a special thanks to the following individual who have spent countless hours and support to make Physeo possible.

Janet E. Lindsley, PhD
Professor, Biochemistry
Assistant Dean, Curriculum
Adjunct Professor, Nutrition and Integrative Physiology
University of Utah School of Medicine

MOLECULAR

Section I - DNA Replication

I. DNA structure (Figure 2.1.1)

A. DNA is complementary to the opposite strand (cytosine pairs with guanine and thymine pairs with adenine).

B. DNA wrapped around eight histones is called a nucleosome.

C. The first histone (H_1) is responsible for linking nucleosomes together.

D. Nucleosomes tightly packed together results in the formation of a chromosome.

1. Tightly packed → heterochromatin (not accessible to transcription proteins)

2. Loosely packed → euchromatin (transcriptionally active)

E. Histone methylation → ↓ DNA transcription

F. Histone acetylation → ↑ DNA transcription

II. DNA replication (Figure 2.1.2)

A. Helicase separates the DNA at the replication fork.

B. Single-stranded binding proteins bind to the DNA and prevent the two strands from reannealing.

C. The region where DNA replication begins is called the origin of replication.

D. Primase anneals to the 3′ end of the DNA and synthesizes a primer.

E. DNA polymerase III binds to the primer and adds deoxynucleotides onto the 3′ end of the primer (eukaryotes perform this function via DNA polymerase epsilon).

1. Synthesizes DNA in the 5′ → 3′ direction.

2. 3′ → 5′ exonuclease activity.

F. The DNA strand being synthesized towards the replication fork is called the leading strand.

1. Synthesized continuously

G. The DNA strand being synthesized away from the replication fork is called the lagging strand.

1. Synthesized discontinuously resulting in the formation of Okazaki fragments.

H. DNA polymerase I (eukaryotes perform removal of primers via DNA polymerase delta) removes the RNA primers and replaces them with DNA.

1. Synthesizes DNA in the 5′ → 3′ direction.

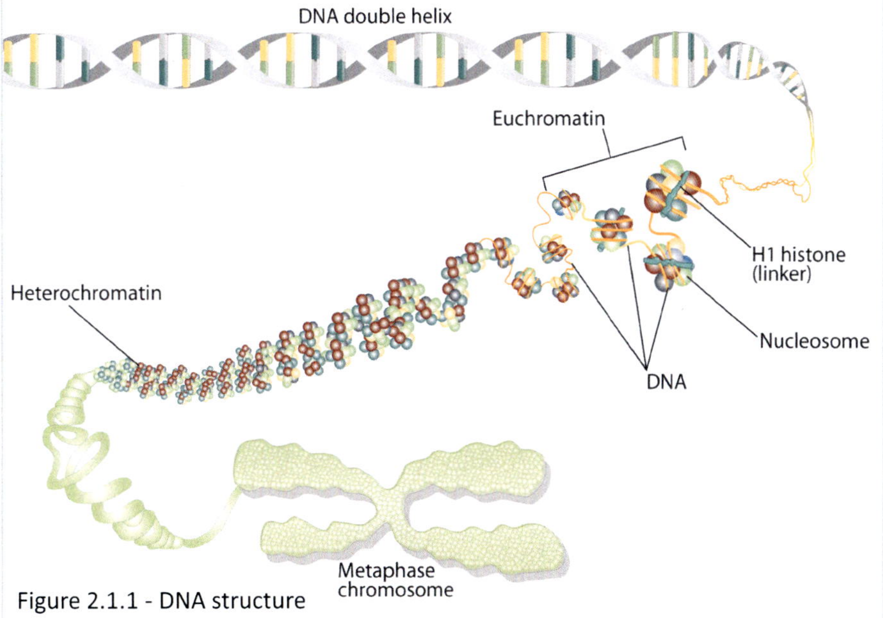

Figure 2.1.1 - DNA structure

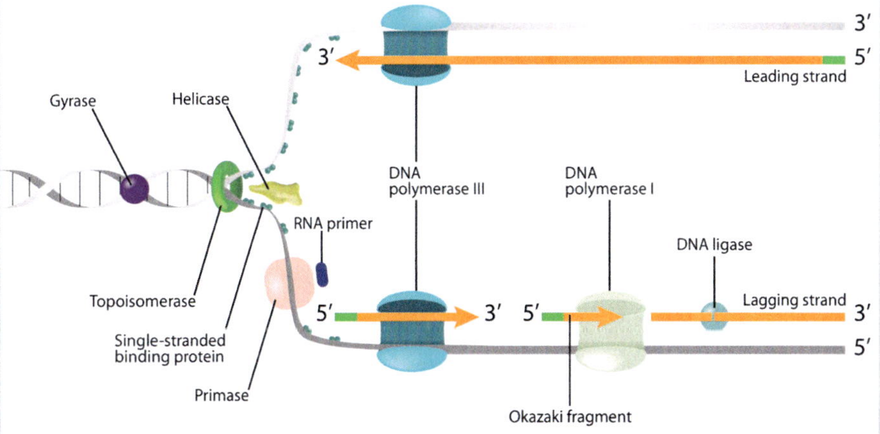

Figure 2.1.2 - DNA replication

2. 5′ → 3′ exonuclease activity.

I. DNA ligase joins the Okazaki fragments

J. Topoisomerases remove supercoils in DNA.

1. Prokaryotic (topoisomerase II & IV)

a) Fluoroquinolones

2. Eukaryotic (topoisomerase I & II)

a) Irinotecan

b) Topotecan

c) Etoposide

d) Teniposide

K. DNA polymerase I vs DNA polymerase III

1. DNA polymerase I ("DNA polymerase I only goes in one direction")

a) 5′ → 3′ synthesis ("contrive at five")

b) 5′ → 3′ exonuclease

L. DNA polymerase III

1. 5′ → 3′ synthesis

2. 3′ → 5′ exonuclease

M. Telomerase

1. Telomere: region at the end of a chromosome

2. Telomerase: enzyme that adds DNA to the 3′ end of chromosomes to prevent the loss of genetic material with every duplication.

REVIEW QUESTIONS ?

1. A new experimental drug is found to inhibit histone deacetylase. How will this drug most likely alter transcription?

- **Acetylation of histones → ↑ transcription**
- **Deacetylation of histones → ↓ transcription**
- **Deacetylase is an enzyme that removes acetyl groups on histones**
- **The drug described inhibits deacetylase → ↑ number of acetylated histones → ↑ transcription**

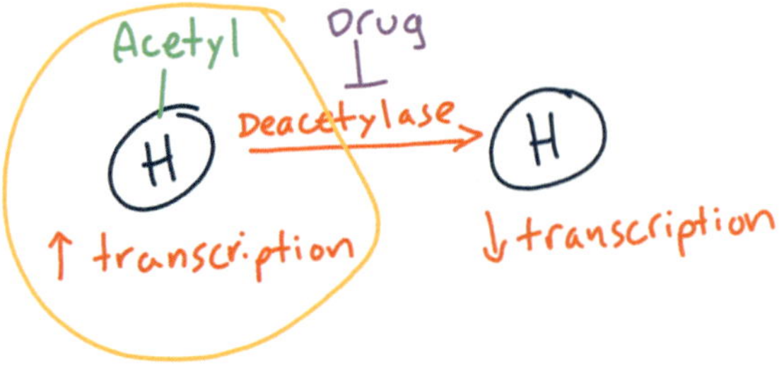

2. A pathologist is studying DNA from staph aureus wound infections. She isolates an enzyme and studies its activity during DNA replication. She finds that this particular enzyme possesses 5′ to 3′ exonuclease activity. What enzyme has she most likely isolated?

- **DNA polymerase I has 5′ to 3′ exonuclease activity**

3. A 76-year-old male is admitted to the hospital for community acquired pneumonia. A sputum culture is obtained in hopes of isolating the pathogen and determining antibiotic sensitivity. As the organism grows, its DNA is extracted and analyzed. Detailed analysis of fragments from partially replicated DNA reveals the presence of ribose sugar molecules with an increased number of hydroxyl modifications. These fragments are most likely degraded by what enzyme during DNA replication?

- **"Detailed analysis of fragments from partially replicated DNA reveals the presence of ribose sugar molecules with an increased number of hydroxyl modifications." → referencing RNA (ribose contains one more hydroxyl group than deoxyribose)**
- **During DNA replication RNA is present in the form of primers**
- **RNA primers are degraded by the enzyme DNA polymerase I**

Section II - DNA Repair

I. Single strand DNA repair

A. Nucleotide excision repair (Figure 2.1.3)

1. Repairs bulky DNA alterations such as pyrimidine dimers (UV radiation).
2. Endonucleases removes nucleotides.
3. DNA polymerase fills in the empty space.
4. Sealed by ligase.
5. Defective in xeroderma pigmentosum.

B. Base excision repair (Figure 2.1.4)

1. Repairs non-bulky DNA alterations such as deamination, depurination, or alkylation (carcinogenic exposure, aging, neurodegeneration).
2. Glycosylase recognizes and cleaves the altered base resulting in an empty sugar-phosphate region known as an apurinic or apyrimidinic (AP) site.
3. Endonuclease cleaves the 5′ end of the AP site.
4. Lyase removes the sugar-phosphate region.
5. DNA polymerase fills in the empty space with the correct sugar.
6. Sealed by ligase.

C. Mismatch repair (Figure 2.1.5)

1. In eukaryotes, replicated DNA is normally proofread by DNA polymerases. However, when this repair mechanism fails, mismatch repair enzymes act as a "backup" repair mechanism.
2. The replicated daughter strand of DNA normally contains nicks in the phosphodiester bonds which distinguishes it from the parent strand of DNA. Two proteins (MutS and MutL) slide along the daughter strand until the nick is found.
3. Exonuclease 1 is recruited to the MutS/MutL complex and degrades a segment of DNA that includes the mismatched base.
4. The gap region is stabilized by single stranded DNA binding proteins.
5. DNA polymerase delta fills in the empty space moving in the 5′ → 3′ direction.
6. Sealed by ligase.
7. Defective in Lynch syndrome (hereditary nonpolyposis colon cancer).

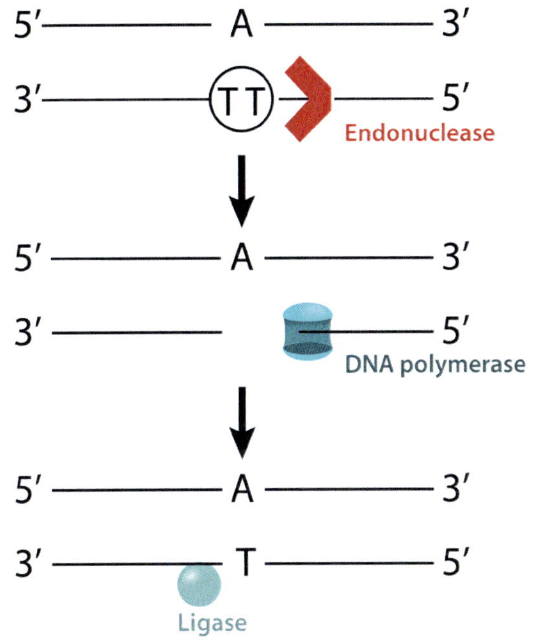

Figure 2.1.3 - Nucleotide excision repair

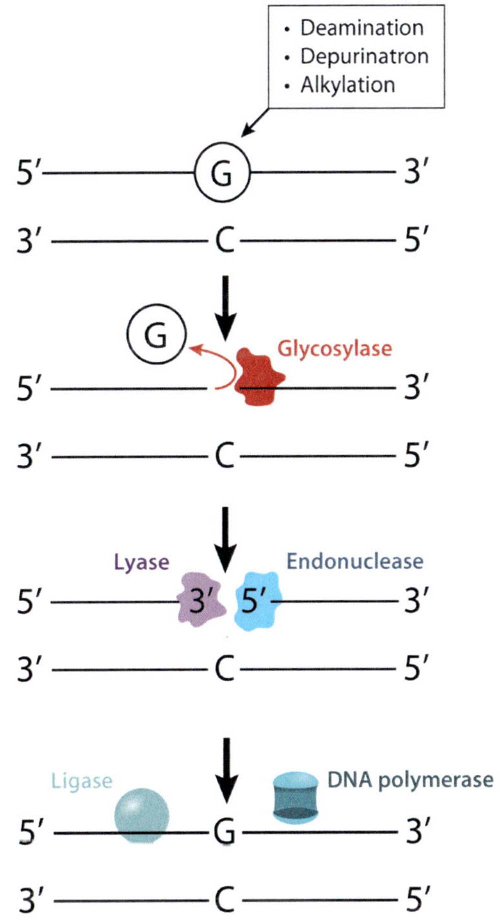

Figure 2.1.4 - Base excision repair

II. Double strand

A. Caused by ionizing radiation

B. Homologous end joining

1. Sister chromosome is used as a template to repair the double stranded break.
2. Associated with Fanconi anemia and gynecological malignancy.

C. Nonhomologous end joining

1. Many proteins required for fixing the broken strands of DNA.
2. Nonhomologous because the sister chromosome is NOT used.
3. ↑ risk of errors
4. Associated with ataxia telangiectasia

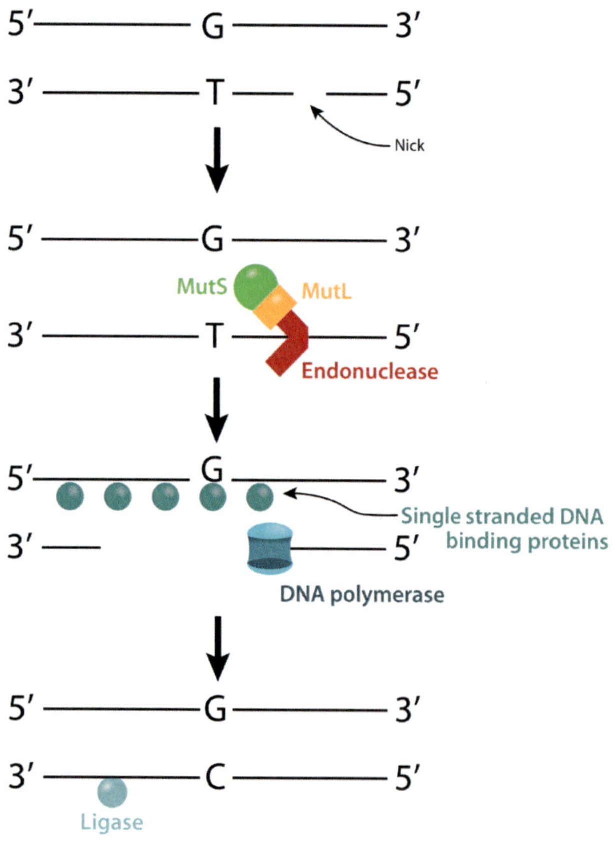

Figure 2.1.5 - Mismatch repair

REVIEW QUESTIONS

1. A 53-year-old male presents with a two month history of cough, fatigue, and weight loss. He endorses a 45-pack-year smoking history. CT scan of the chest reveals an irregular mass near the inferior lobe of the right lung. Biopsy samples are obtained. Further analysis reveals malignant cells with heavily alkylated regions of DNA. What are the first three enzymes normally associated with repairing this type of damaged DNA?

   - **This patient has lung cancer and the malignant cells contain heavily alkylated regions of DNA**
   - **Base excision repair is responsible for repairing non-bulky DNA alterations (deamination, depurination, or alkylation)**
   - **Carcinogenic exposure (i.e. smoking) can cause non-bulky DNA alterations**
   - **Glycosylase, endonuclease, and lyase are the first three enzymes associated with base excision repair**

2. A 40-year-old female presents with two months of bloody vaginal discharge. She states that her cycle normally occurs every 28 days and flow normally lasts 3-4 days. Two years ago she had an ovarian malignancy surgically removed. The physician confirms a diagnosis of endometrial carcinoma. However, he suspects a genetic condition as the underlying cause and orders a fecal occult blood test which comes back positive. DNA analysis of malignant tissue would most likely reveal cytosine-rich regions of DNA pairing with what other base?

   - **Ovarian, endometrial, and likely colon cancer (positive fecal occult blood test) → Lynch syndrome**
   - **Lynch syndrome is due to mutations of DNA mismatch repair genes**
   - **Normally cytosine pairs with guanine**
   - **A defect in mismatch repair → cytosine abnormally paired with adenine and thymine rather than guanine**

Section III - Transcription

I. Overview (Figure 2.1.6)

A. Transcription is a process whereby mRNA is synthesized using DNA as a template.

B. Prokaryotes: DNA → mRNA → protein

C. Eukaryotes: DNA → pre-mRNA → mature mRNA → protein

D. Promoter: located before the gene and facilitates the binding of RNA polymerase to this region

E. Enhancer: increases the rate of transcription

F. Silencer: decreases the rate of transcription

II. Transcription (Figure 2.1.7)

A. RNA polymerase binds to the promoter region.

1. Eukaryotes have three types of RNA polymerases

a) RNA polymerase I: rRNA (nucleolus)

b) RNA polymerase II: mRNA (inhibited by amatoxins)

c) RNA polymerase III: tRNA and other RNA

2. Prokaryotes

a) One RNA polymerase performs all functions (inhibited by antibiotics)

B. Pre-mRNA is synthesized in the 5′ → 3′ direction from the template strand of DNA.

C. A molecule of modified guanine is added to the 5′ end of the pre-mRNA (5′ cap).

D. Several adenine molecules are added to the 3′ end of the pre-mRNA (poly-A tail).

E. The introns are removed through a process known as splicing to form mature mRNA.

III. Splicing

A. Introns are removed by structures called spliceosomes.

1. Small nuclear ribonucleoproteins (snRNPs) + protein = spliceosome.

B. The intron nucleotides directly adjacent to the exons are important for proper splicing.

C. An intermediate intron structure is formed called a Lariat intermediate.

D. Alternative splicing is a process whereby one gene may produce multiple types of mature mRNA molecules and ultimately multiple types of proteins.

IV. RNA interference is a process whereby specific types of RNA sequences induce gene silencing (mRNA that has already been transcribed is destroyed).

A. MicroRNA (miRNA)

1. Double-stranded pre-miRNA transcribed in nucleus

2. A ribonuclease protein (dicer) in the cytosol cleaves the pre-miRNA → mature miRNA

3. Mature miRNA combines with proteins → RNA-induced silencing complex (RISC)

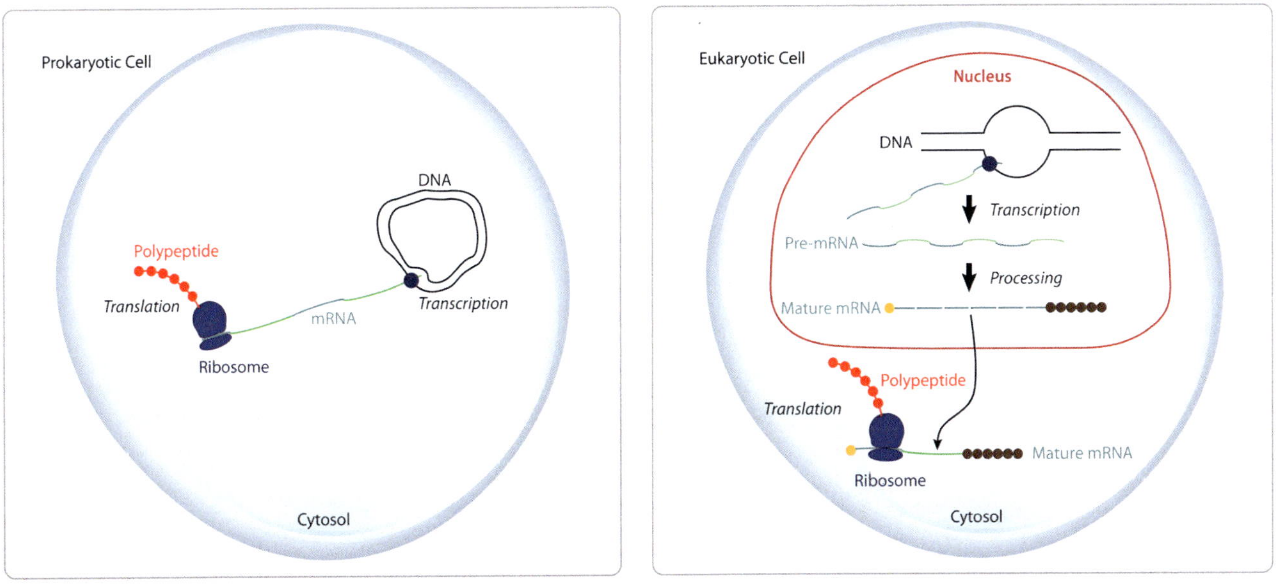

Figure 2.1.6 - Transcription and translation overview

4. The miRNA template of the RISC can bind to complementary sequences of mRNA → degradation

B. Small interfering RNA (siRNA) is a synthetically produced RNA with similar functionality to miRNA. (Figure 2.1.8)

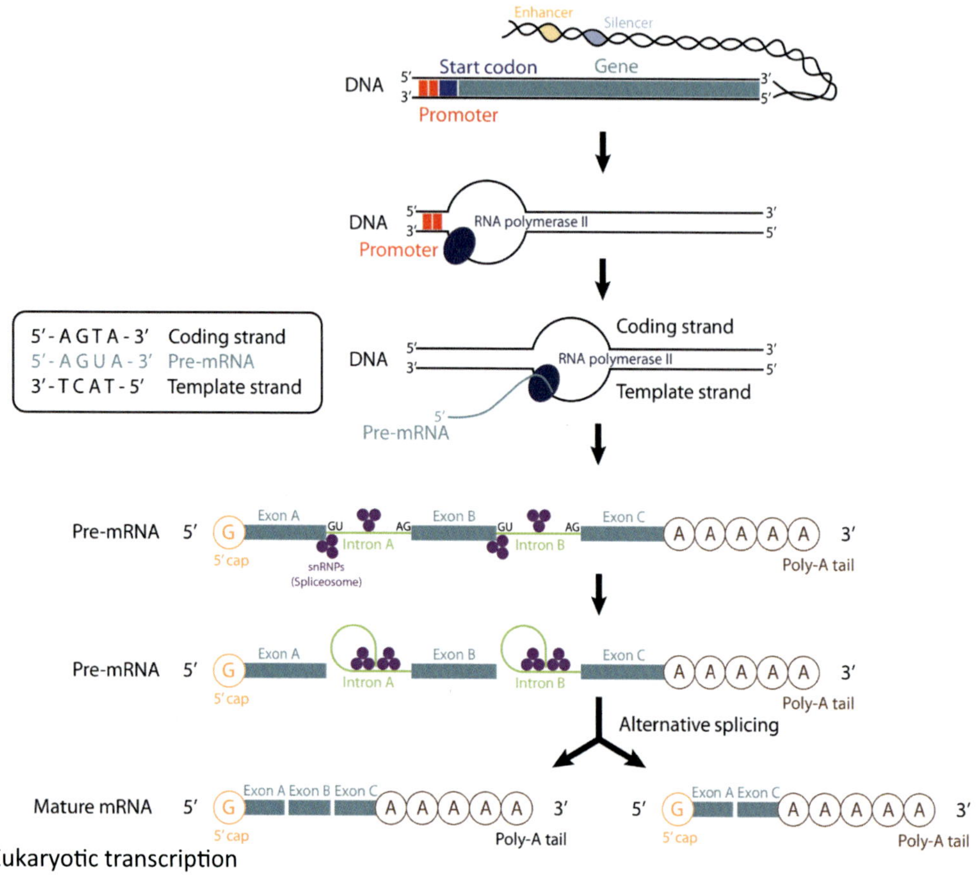

Figure 2.1.7 - Eukaryotic transcription

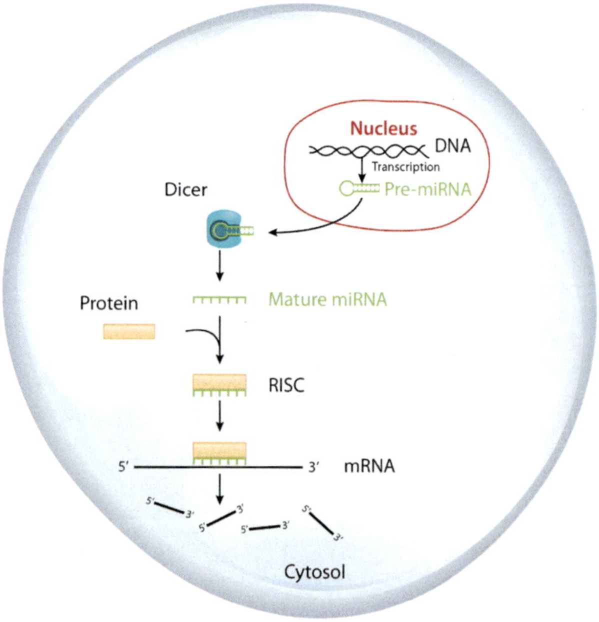

Figure 2.1.8 - RNA interference

REVIEW QUESTIONS

1. Why do the malignant cells shown below have prominent nucleoli?

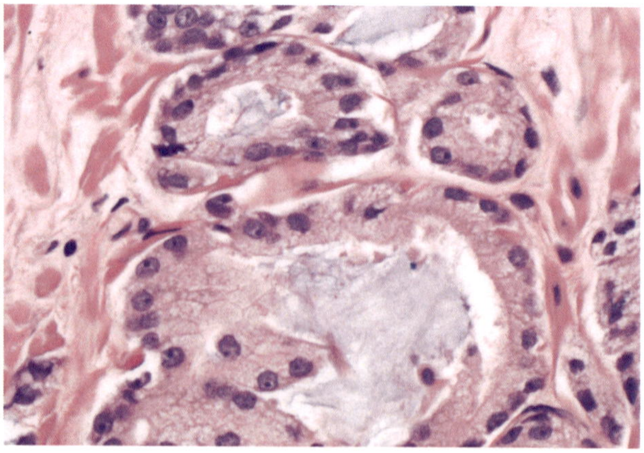

- **The nucleolus is the site of synthesis and assembly of rRNA**
- **Malignant cells are very active → ↑ protein synthesis → ↑ transcription of rRNA → darkening of nucleoli**

REVIEW QUESTIONS

2. A 12-year-old girl presents with a facial rash, joint pain, and a fever. Laboratory analysis reveals the presence of anti-Smith antibodies. A sequence of pre-mRNA is obtained from the patient. The highlighted region represents an intron and the non-highlighted regions are exons.

5'-GUAACGUAAGUACGCGAGAGAGAACAGCA
UACGUAAGUAACGUAAGUACGCGAGAGAGU
GAUGGAGAUGGAGAUGGAGAUGGAGAUGG
AGAUGGAGAUGGAGAUGGAGACGUAAGUA-
CGCGAGAGAGAACAGCAUACGUAAGUAACG-
UAAGUACGCGAGAGAACAGCAGGCGGGC-3'

The antibodies described above bind to a structure that normally binds to the intron. What colored region in the intron shown above does this structure most likely rely upon for proper splicing?

- **Facial rash, joint pain, fever, anti-Smith antibodies → lupus**
- **"The antibodies described above bind to a structure that normally binds to the intron" → referring to spliceosome**
- **Anti-Smith antibodies bind to snRNPs (spliceosome consists of snRNPs + protein)**
- **The red regions (GU and AG) are regions in the intron directly adjacent to the exons and are important for proper splicing**

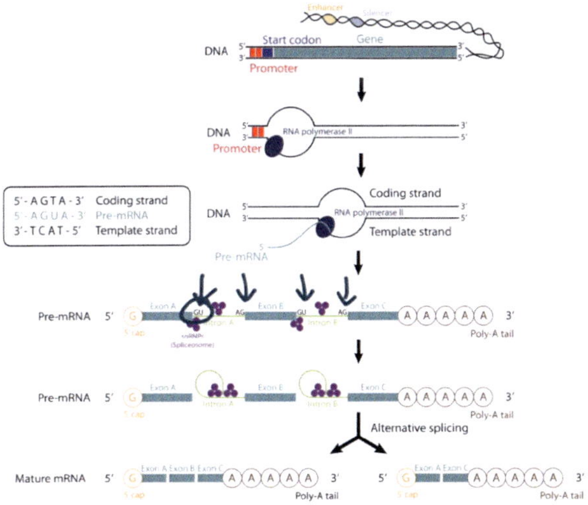

3. A 19-year-old male presents to the ED with vomiting, diarrhea, and abdominal pain. He was emergently driven to the hospital from a nearby trail where he ingested some wild mushrooms. What laboratory findings would most likely be present in this patient?

- **Wild mushrooms may contain amatoxins → inhibition of RNA polymerase II (synthesizes mRNA)**
- **Toxins are ingested → transported to liver → ↓ hepatic mRNA synthesis → apoptosis → ↑ AST & ALT**

4. A pharmaceutical company has developed a treatment for Alzheimer disease. Normally the amyloid precursor protein (APP) gene is transcribed into mRNA which ultimately results in the production of amyloid beta peptides. Overproduction of these peptides are thought to be the cause of Alzheimer disease. In several clinical trials, this new drug was shown to decrease the levels of mature mRNA transcribed from the APP gene. However, the levels of pre-mRNA transcribed from the APP gene were elevated. Based on the information above, what can most likely be deduced about the mechanism of action of the newly developed drug?

- **The drug ↓ the levels of mature mRNA but the levels of pre-mRNA remain elevated**
- **The drug is most likely siRNA (synthetically derived miRNA)**
- **siRNA destroys mRNA**

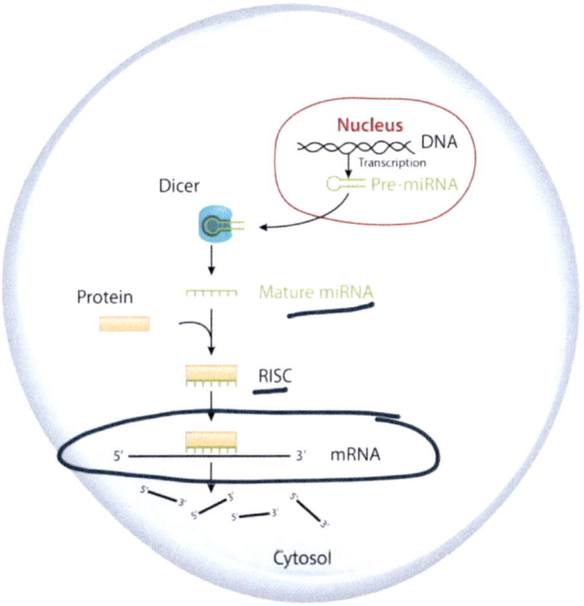

Section IV - Translation

I. Translation is a process whereby polypeptides are synthesized using mRNA as a template. (Figure 2.1.9)

II. Transfer ribonucleic acid (tRNA) is a molecule that transfers amino acids to the growing polypeptide.

A. D-arm (binds aminoacyl tRNA synthetase)

B. T-arm (binds ribosome)

C. Anticodon loop (contains anticodon that pairs with the codon in mRNA)

1. Sometimes the anticodon in a tRNA molecule is still able to pair with an mRNA codon even if the bases do not perfectly complement one another, a process known as wobble pairing.

D. Acceptor site (binds amino acids)

E. Aminoacyl tRNA synthetase is the enzyme responsible for combining a molecule of tRNA with an amino acid (charging).

III. Ribosomes

A. A site: accepts charged tRNA

B. P site: tRNA is processed (polypeptide formation)

C. E site: tRNA exits

D. Differences in eukaryotic and prokaryotic ribosomal structure allow antibiotics to specifically target prokaryotic ribosomes while sparing eukaryotic ribosomes.

IV. Polypeptide synthesis

A. Initiation

1. Initiation factors and GTP are used to bring the large and small subunits together along with mRNA and tRNA.

2. The Kozak sequence is a region next to the start codon that facilitates the binding of the small ribosomal subunit to the mRNA.

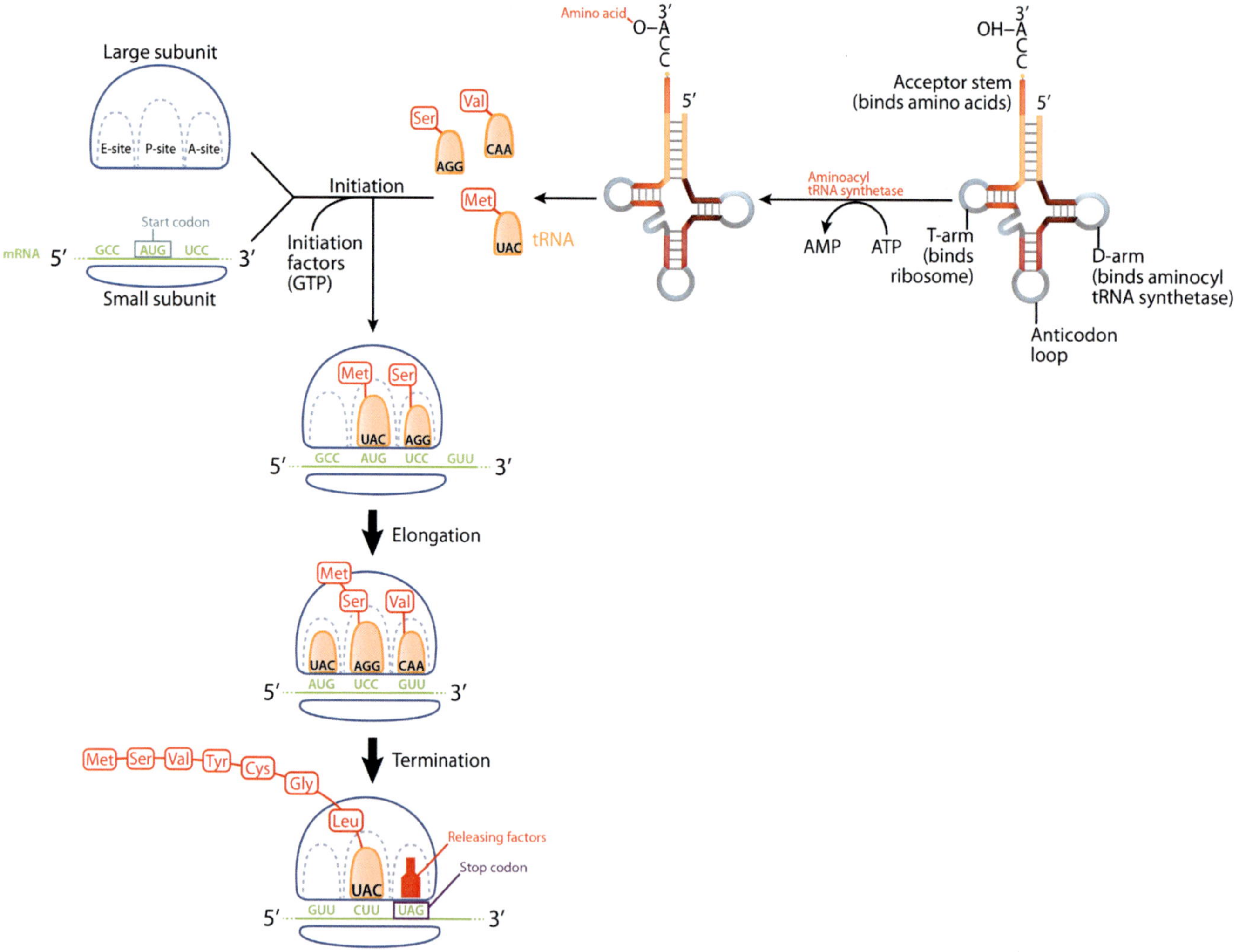

Figure 2.1.9 - Translation

3. The start codon is usually AUG ("AUG inAUGurates protein synthesis"). Rarely, the start codon may be GUG.

B. Elongation

1. The tRNA and mRNA molecules move through the ribosomes resulting in a growing polypeptide.
2. mRNA is read in the 5′ to 3′ direction.
3. Specific elongation factors are required for this step to occur (i.e. EF-2).

C. Termination

1. A stop codon (UGA, UAA, UAG) in the mRNA is encountered
   a) "UGA = U Go Away"
   b) "UAA = U Are Away"
   c) "UAG = U Are Gone"
2. Releasing factors (do not contain amino acids) bind to the ribosome at the stop codon site → dissociation of ribosomal complex

D. Posttranslational modifications (methylation, acetylation, etc.) can occur after translation.

REVIEW QUESTIONS

1. Researchers are studying the process of translation in mice. In one particular mouse model, a knockout mutation results in embryonic demise. Upon further analysis the researchers discover that the mutation results in modified bases inserted at the 3′ end of the molecules normally responsible for binding amino acids. They also notice that in this particular mouse model the activity of aminoacyl tRNA synthetase is decreased. What is the most likely normal composition of the 3′ end of the mutated molecule?

- **"Molecule normally responsible for binding amino acids" → referring to tRNA**
- **The 3′ end contains the base sequence CCA**

REVIEW QUESTIONS

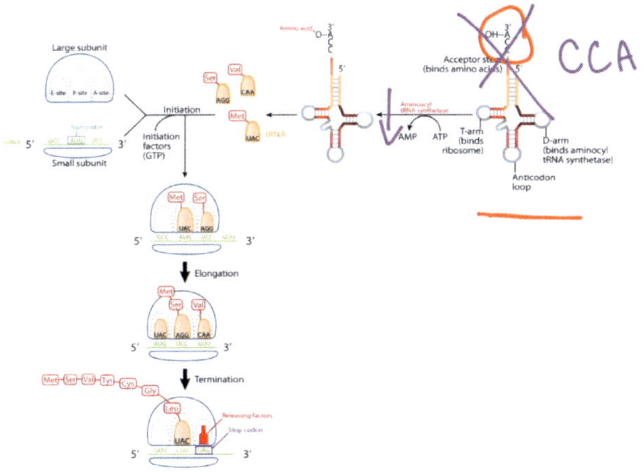

2. A 7-year-old unimmunized boy presents with a sore throat that started three days ago. He has also noticed malaise and low-grade fevers. On exam he has cervical lymphadenopathy, pharyngeal erythema, and coalescing patches of gray fibrotic tissue directly adjacent to his tonsils. The physician suspects that this patient's symptoms are due to an infectious organism that produces an exotoxin. This exotoxin most likely inhibits what factor associated with eukaryotic translation?

- **Pharyngitis and coalescing patches of gray fibrotic tissue (pseudomembrane) → corynebacterium diphtheriae**
- **Corynebacterium diphtheriae produces diphtheria toxin (an exotoxin) → inhibits elongation factor 2 (EF-2)**

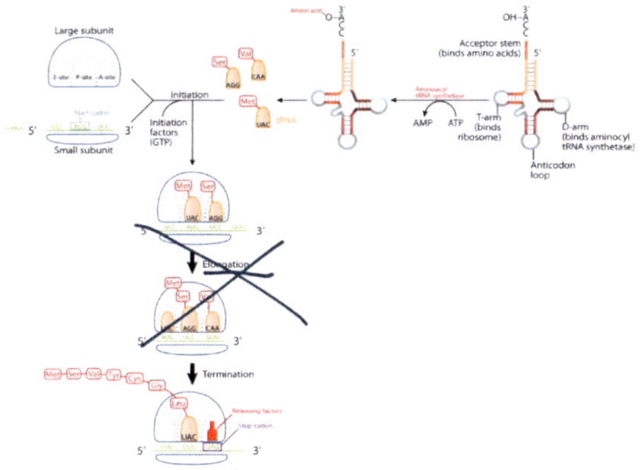

Section V - DNA Mutations

Second letter

First letter	U	C	A	G	Third letter
U	UUU, UUC – Phe UUA, UUG – Leu	UCU, UCC, UCA, UCG – Leu	UAU, UAC – Tyr UAA – Stop UAG – Stop	UGU, UGC – Cys UGA – Stop UGG – Trp	U C A G
C	CUU, CUC, CUA, CUG – Leu	CCU, CCC, CCA, CCG – Pro	CAU, CAC – His CAA, CAG – Gln	CGU, CGC, CGA, CGG – Arg	U C A G
A	AUU, AUC, AUA – Ile AUG – Met (start)	ACU, ACC, ACA, ACG – Thr	AAU, AAC – Asn AAA, AAG – Lys	AGU, AGC – Ser AGA, AGG – Arg	U C A G
G	GUU, GUC, GUA, GUG – Val	GCU, GCC, GCA, GCG – Ala	GAU, GAC – Asp GAA, GAG – Glu	GGU, GGC, GGA, GGG – Gly	U C A G

Figure 2.1.10 - Genetic code

Mutation	Description	Example
Silent	Caused by nucleotide substitutions that do not result in a different amino acid	ACC (Thr) → ACG (Thr)
Missense	Caused by nucleotide substitutions that result in a different amino acid	ACC (Thr) → AAC (Asn)
Nonsense	Caused by nucleotide substitutions that result in a premature stop codon	UAC (Tyr) → UAG (STOP)
Frameshift	Caused by insertions or deletions that cause a shift in the reading frame such that many amino acids are coded for incorrectly	See corresponding figure
DNA slippage	Caused by a segment of DNA that slips away from the complementary strand → frameshift mutations	See corresponding figure
Splice site	Caused by mutations in regions associated with the splicing of pre-mRNA and results in retained introns	See corresponding figure

DNA	3′	TAA	TCG	ATG	5′
mRNA	5′	AUU	AGC	ACC	3′
Amino acids		Ile	Ser	Thr	

↓ Frameshift mutation

DNA	3′	(A)TA	ATC	GAT	G . . . 5′
mRNA	5′	UAU	UAG	CAC	3′
Amino acids		Tyr	STOP	His	

Figure 2.1.11 - Frameshift mutations

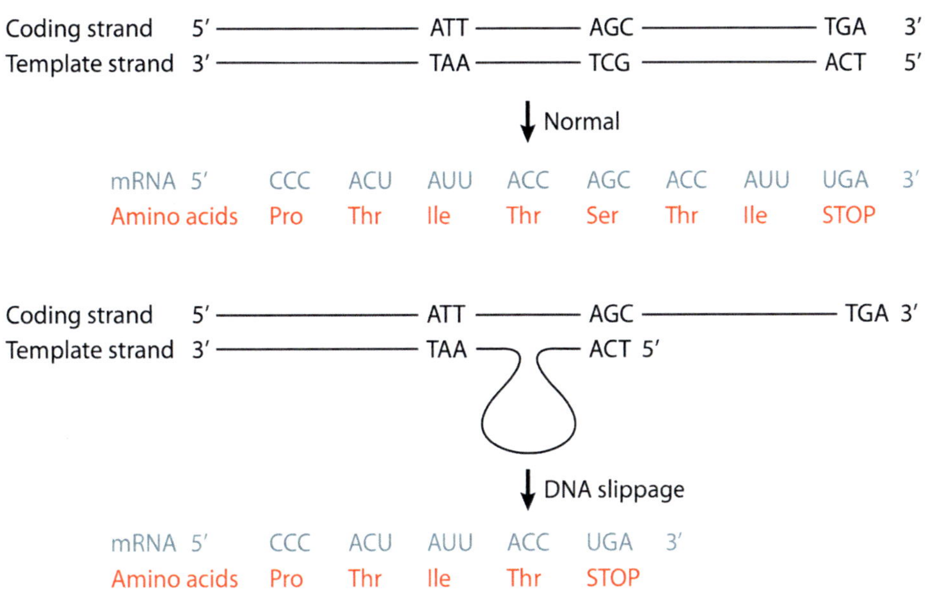

Figure 2.1.12 - DNA slippage

REVIEW QUESTIONS

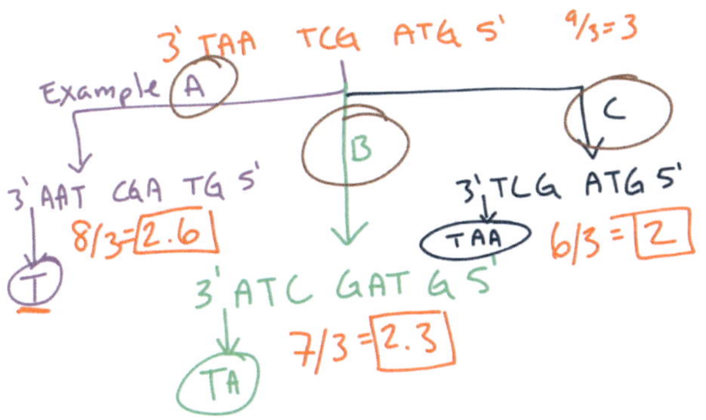

1. A 5-year-old boy is being evaluated for Duchenne muscular dystrophy. Laboratory analysis reveals a mutated mRNA molecule. The molecule is reverse transcribed into cDNA which is found to be 976 bases shorter than a control group. What genetic defect is most likely responsible for this patient's condition?

   A) Silent mutation
   B) Missense mutation
   C) Nonsense mutation
   D) Frameshift mutation

- **976 base pair deletion**
- **976 is not divisible by 3 → frameshift mutation (these are not divisible by 3)**
- **The patient most likely has a frameshift mutation**
- **Nonsense mutations are divisible by 3**

2. A segment of the β-globin gene is shown below. The capital letters represent exons and the lowercase letters represent introns. A mutation region shown below would most likely result in β-thalassemia?

5′-TGCGCAACCGGATGgtattgccggaatagatgcgatgaagt
gcaccgaggctgagGGAACCTGAGTCGAGCTAGACG
gtactagtatattttaaccgactgagtacaggaagGGGGAACCT
TAGGGATTAGCGAGTGACCCAC-3′

   A) G (yellow)
   B) a (orange)
   C) T (green)
   D) C (red)

- **Only choice B represents a mutated intron**
- **Mutations in the introns are a common cause of β-thalassemia (a genetic disorder resulting in abnormal hemoglobin)**
- **B-thalassemia can also be caused by mutations to the promoter region**

CELLULAR

Section I - Cell Cycle

I. Cell cycle phases (Figure 2.2.1)

A. Interphase

1. G_0 - a non-dividing resting state
2. G_1 - first growth phase (synthesis of carbohydrates, proteins, lipids, and RNA)
3. S - DNA synthesized
4. G_2 - second growth phase (synthesis of ATP)

B. Mitosis (M)

1. Prophase: chromosomes condense and spindle fibers form.
2. Metaphase: chromosomes line up in the middle of cell.
3. Anaphase: chromosomes separate to opposite sides of the cell.
4. Telophase: the cell divides and replicated chromosomes are equally split among daughter cells.

II. Cell types

A. Permanent - always in G_0

1. Muscle cells, neurons, and RBCs

B. Stable (quiescent) - alternate between G_0 and G_1

1. Hepatocytes and lymphocytes

C. Labile - rapidly dividing and rarely in G_0

1. Bone marrow cells, skin, hair follicles, and gut epithelial cells

III. Cell cycle regulation (Figure 2.2.2)

A. Cyclins bind cyclin dependent kinases (CDKs) → cyclin-CDK complex → phosphorylation (inactivation) of retinoblastoma protein (Rb) → release of E2F (transcription factor) → cellular division

B. Cyclin D1 promotes cell cycle progression (G_1 → S) and dysregulation is implicated in mantle cell lymphoma

C. Abnormal Rb protein is implicated in retinoblastoma

D. Li-Fraumeni syndrome is caused by mutations in p53

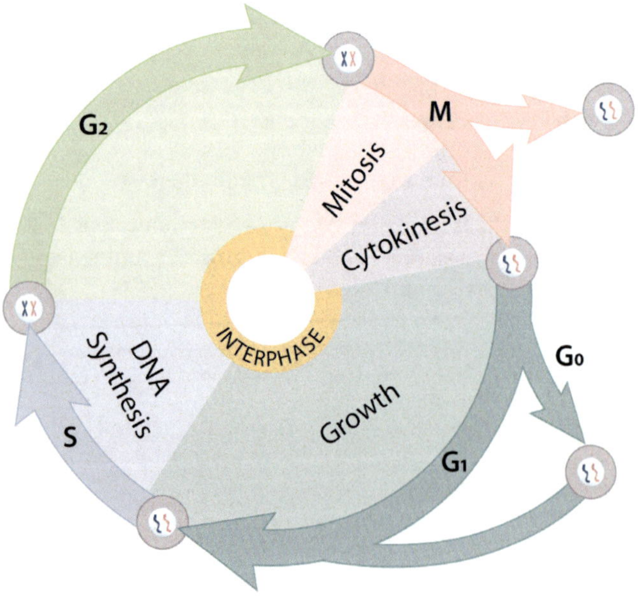

Figure 2.2.1 - Cell cycle

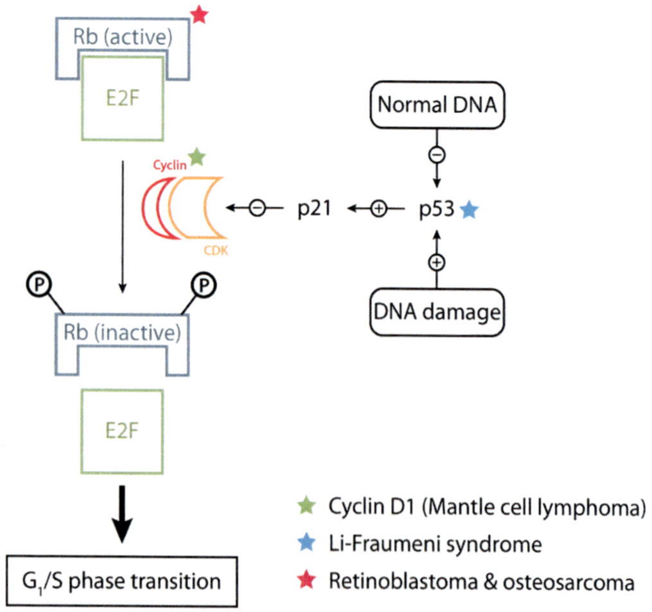

Figure 2.2.2 - Regulation of G1/S phase transition

REVIEW QUESTIONS

1. Researchers are studying the effects of a new drug on the cell cycle in mice. The mice are exposed to the new drug and then several proteins are isolated. One protein of interest is found to be heavily phosphorylated by the new drug, resulting in an altered interaction with the transcription factor E2F. How would the activity of DNA polymerase III likely be altered as a result of exposure to the new drug?

   - **The new drug increases the phosphorylation of a protein (Rb) → release of E2F → G_1/S phase transition → ↑ DNA synthesis → ↑ DNA polymerase III**

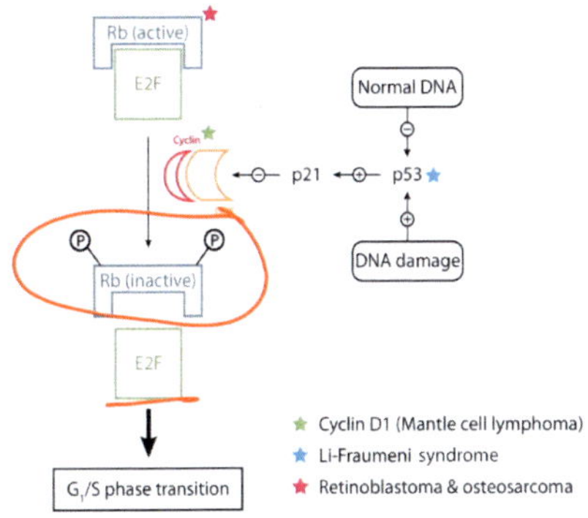

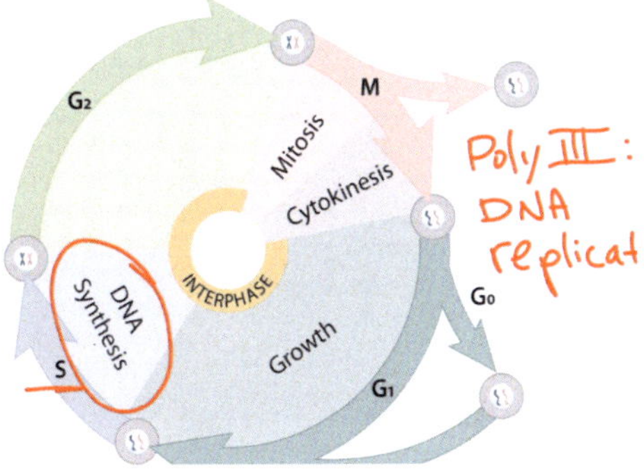

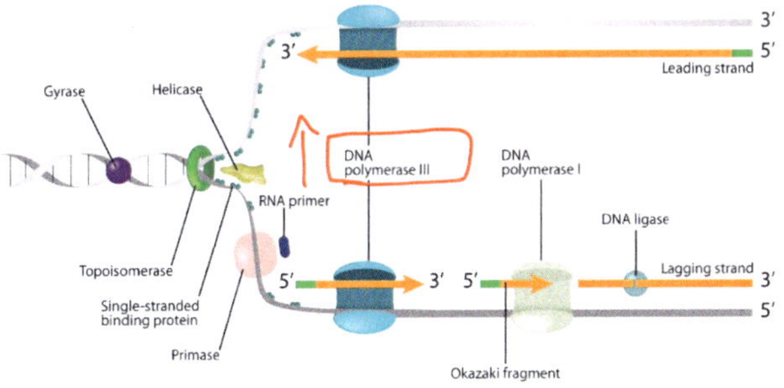

2. A 12-year-old girl presents to the office for a follow up visit. She has a history of xeroderma pigmentosum and requires frequent visits to screen for skin cancer. How will the activity of p53 likely be altered in this patient?

   - **Xeroderma pigmentosum → ↓ nucleotide excision repair → ↑ DNA damage → ↑ p53**

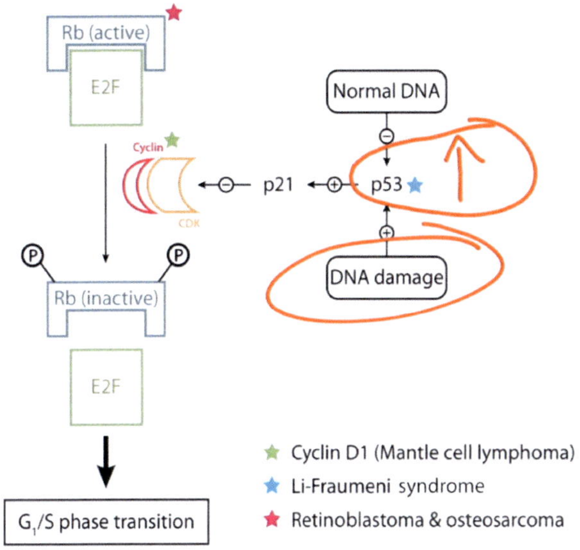

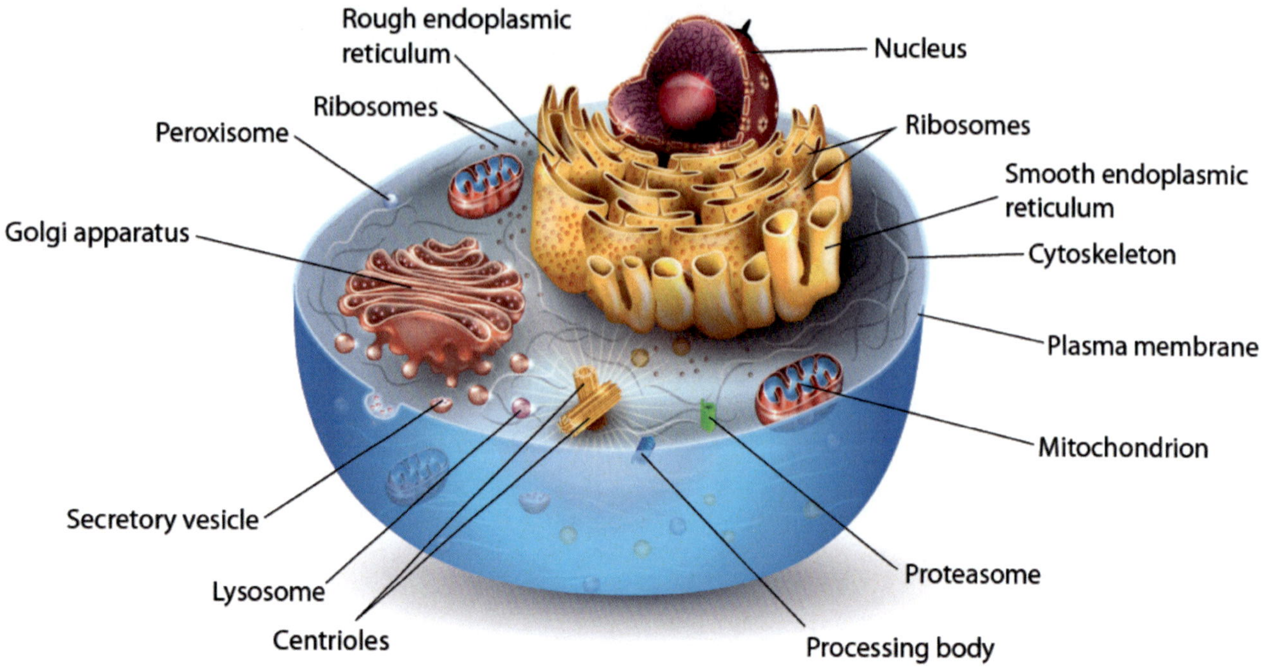

Figure 2.2.3 - Cell anatomy

Structure	Function	Notes
Nucleus	- Stores DNA	
Rough endoplasmic reticulum (RER)	- Synthesis of proteins that will be exported to outside of cell (peptide hormones)	- Nissl bodies (RER in neurons)
Smooth endoplasmic reticulum (SER)	- Site of lipid and steroid synthesis (steroid hormones)	
Golgi apparatus	- Modifies proteins and transports to target location	- Phosphorylation of mannose on proteins → lysosomes - I cell disease
Processing bodies (p-bodies)	- Regulation of mRNA	
Mitochondria	- Generation of ATP	
Lysosome	- Breakdown obsolete components of cell	- Lysosomal storage diseases
Peroxisome	- Oxidize very long and branched chain fatty acids - Perform hydrogen peroxide degradation (catalase)	- X-linked adrenoleukodystrophy - Zellweger syndrome
Proteasome	- Degrades proteins marked by ubiquitin	- Parkinson disease - Alzheimer disease
Microfilament (actin)	- Muscle contraction (sarcomere) - Nutrient absorption (microvilli) - Cell structure (adherens junction)	
Intermediate filament	- Cell structure - Immunohistochemical staining of these filaments used to identify tumors	- Keratin (epithelium - squamous cell carcinoma) - Desmin (muscle - rhabdomyosarcoma) - Vimentin (mesenchymal tissue - sarcoma) - GFAP (neuroglia - astrocytoma) - Neurofilaments (neurons - neuroblastoma)
Microtubule	- Cell motility (flagella, cilia) - Intracellular transportation (neurotransmitters) - Mitosis (mitotic spindle)	- Kartagener's syndrome - Blocked by many drugs (vincristine, paclitaxel, griseofulvin)

Table 2.2.1 - Cell Structure and Function

I. I-cell disease

A. Defect in N-acetylglucosaminyl-1-phosphotransferase

B. Proteins are secreted rather than delivered to lysosomes

C. Symptoms include coarse facial features, failure to thrive, cognitive impairment, and corneal clouding

II. Cell trafficking (Figure 2.2.4)

A. Vesicles can be coated with various proteins

1. Clathrin (between Golgi apparatus and plasma membrane)

2. COPI (Golgi → endoplasmic reticulum)

3. COPII (endoplasmic reticulum → golgi)

III. Peroxisomal diseases

A. Zellweger syndrome

1. Defective peroxisome function → ↑ very long chain fatty acids (VLCFAs)

B. X-linked adrenoleukodystrophy

1. Impaired transport of VLCFAs to peroxisomes → ↑ VLCFAs in brain (cognitive impairment) and adrenal glands (adrenal insufficiency)

IV. Kartagener's syndrome

A. Defective dynein arm → immotile cilia

B. Infertility (men and women)

C. ↑ risk of ectopic pregnancy (women)

D. Bronchiectasis

E. Situs inversus

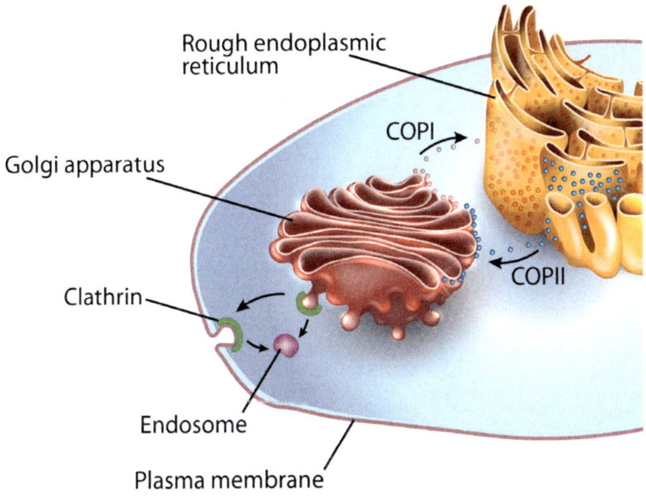

Figure 2.2.4 - Cell trafficking

REVIEW QUESTIONS

1. A 24-year-old female presents to the physician with concerns regarding breast milk production. She states that she has never been pregnant and has no children. She also notes that her breasts have enlarged over the past several months and she recently began producing milk. On exam she is noted to have bitemporal hemianopsia. Her presentation is most consistent with a disorder caused by overproduction of a hormone produced by what cellular organelle?

- **Galactorrhea and bitemporal hemianopsia → prolactinoma**
- **Prolactin is a peptide hormone (synthesized in rough endoplasmic reticulum)**

2. A 7-month-old boy is brought to the physician due to failure to thrive and cognitive delay. Upon further analysis the boy is discovered to have impaired transportation of proteins to an organelle that is normally responsible for degrading obsolete components of the cell. What specific carbohydrate normally found on the proteins described above is most likely deficient in this individual?

- **"Impaired transportation of proteins to an organelle that is normally responsible for degrading obsolete components of the cell" → organelle described is a lysosome**
- **The Golgi apparatus normally send proteins to lysosomes**
- **This patient has I cell disease (a lysosomal storage disease caused by defective phosphorylation of mannose residues in the Golgi apparatus)**
- **Phosphorylation of mannose sugar molecules results in mannose-6-phosphate (acts as a signal for the protein to go to the lysosome)**
- **The patient most likely has ↓ mannose-6-phosphate residues found on proteins**

3. A 12-year-old female presents with a non-tender slowly enlarging mass near the left orbit. Biopsy of the mass reveals poorly differentiated cells that stain positive for desmin. What is the most likely origin of the cells seen on the biopsy?

A) Epithelial cells
B) Muscle cells
C) Mesenchymal tissue
D) Neurons

- **Desmin is an intermediate filament present in muscle cells → answer is B**
- **Rhabdomyosarcoma is the most likely diagnosis**

Section III - Connective tissue

I. Overview

A. Connective tissue is an abundant supportive tissue throughout the body.

B. Three important components of connective tissue include collagen, elastin, and fibrillin.

II. Collagen

A. Most abundant protein in the body

B. Found in bone, skin, cartilage, blood vessels, and others

C. Types I-IV

D. Associated with scurvy, osteogenesis imperfecta, Ehlers-Danlos syndrome, and Menkes disease.

III. Collagen synthesis (Figure 2.2.5)

A. Collagen is synthesized by chondroblasts, osteoblasts, and fibroblasts.

B. In the rough endoplasmic reticulum, the pro-α-chain is synthesized which consists of a repetitive amino acid sequence (glycine-X-Y; X & Y = proline or lysine).

C. Hydroxylation occurs (requires vitamin C; deficiency → scurvy).

D. Glycosylation occurs

E. Assembly of pro-α-chains into procollagen (defects → osteogenesis imperfecta)

F. Procollagen peptidases cleave C- & N- terminal peptides (defect → Ehlers-Danlos syndrome)

1. Procollagen is transferred from the Golgi apparatus to the extracellular space where the terminal C- and N- terminal propeptides are cleaved by procollagen peptidases.

G. Cross-linking occurs via lysyl oxidase → formation of strong collagen fibers (decreased activity of lysyl oxidase → Menkes disease; Ehlers-Danlos syndrome)

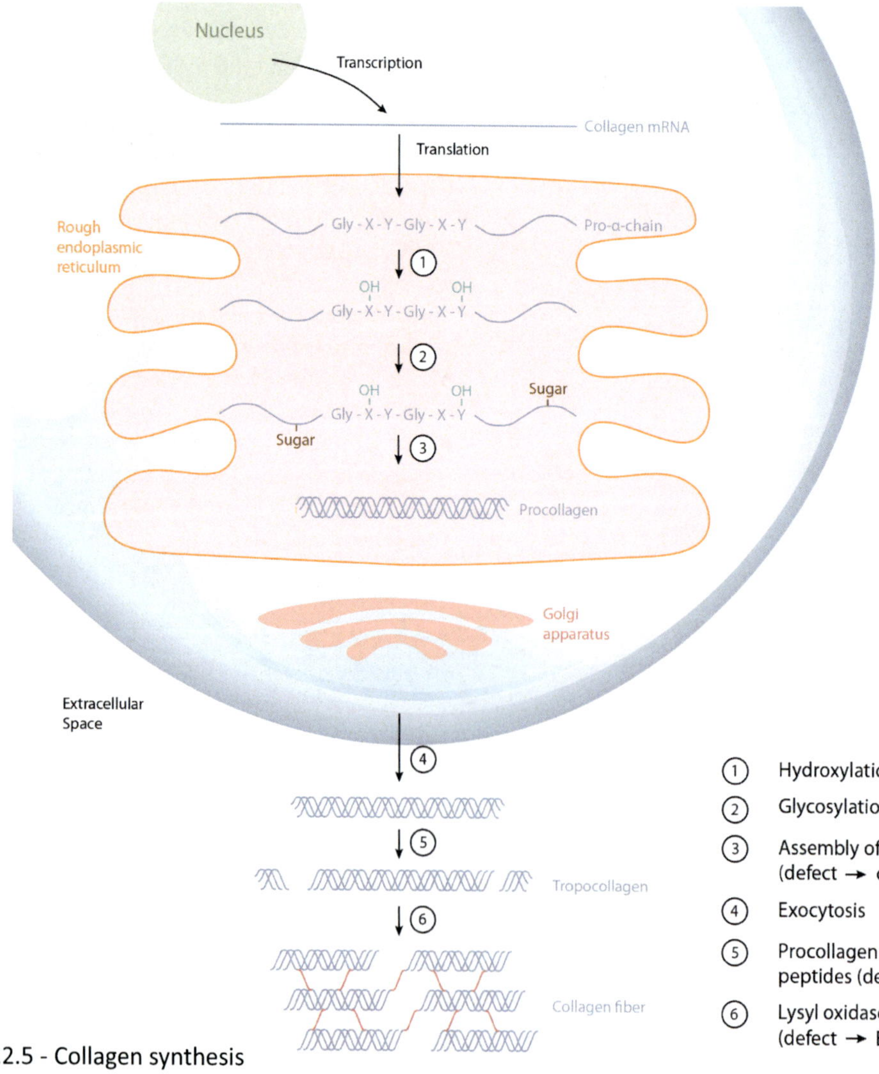

(1) Hydroxylation (requires vitamin C; defect → scurvy)
(2) Glycosylation
(3) Assembly of pro-α-chains into procollagen (defect → osteogenesis imperfecta)
(4) Exocytosis
(5) Procollagen peptidases cleave C-terminal & N-terminal peptides (defect → Ehlers-Danlos syndrome)
(6) Lysyl oxidase (copper cofactor) cross-links molecules (defect → Ehlers-Danlos syndrome; Menkes disease)

Figure 2.2.5 - Collagen synthesis

IV. Scurvy

A. ↓ fruits and vegetables → vitamin C deficiency → ↓ collagen hydroxylation → ↓ collagen synthesis and connective tissue strength

B. Clinical features

1. Swollen gums
2. Poor wound healing
3. Bruising

V. Osteogenesis imperfecta

A. Autosomal dominant genetic disorder (COL1A1 and COL1A2 genes)

B. ↓ formation of procollagen → ↓ collagen

C. Clinical features

1. Multiple fractures (may be confused with abuse),
2. Blue sclerae (translucent connective tissue → choroidal veins become more prominent),
3. Hearing loss (ossicles),
4. Abnormal teeth

VI. Ehlers-Danlos syndrome

A. Deficiency of procollagen peptidase or lysyl oxidase

B. ↓ cross-linked collagen → weaker and more elastic

C. Classic type

1. Stretchy skin
2. Easy bruising
3. Hypermobile joints

D. Vascular type

1. CNS aneurysms

VII. Menkes disease

A. ↓ copper absorption → lysyl oxidase → ↓ cross-linked collagen

B. Growth retardation

C. Brittle hair

D. Hypotonia

VIII. Elastin synthesis (Figure 2.2.6)

A. Synthesis is similar to collagen

B. Elastin is dependent on a scaffold of microfibril molecules

C. Fibrillin-1 is a component of microfibrils (defects → Marfan syndrome)

D. Lysyl oxidase cross-linking in collagen synthesis results in strong collagen. In elastin synthesis, however, this contributes to the elastic and stretchy property of elastin.

IX. Marfan syndrome

A. Defects in fibrillin-1 → microfibril scaffold for elastin disrupted → weak connective tissue

B. Abundant in heart, lens, and periosteum

C. Features include aortic dissection, mitral valve prolapse, cataracts, Marfanoid habitus (tall with long extremities), and pectus excavatum

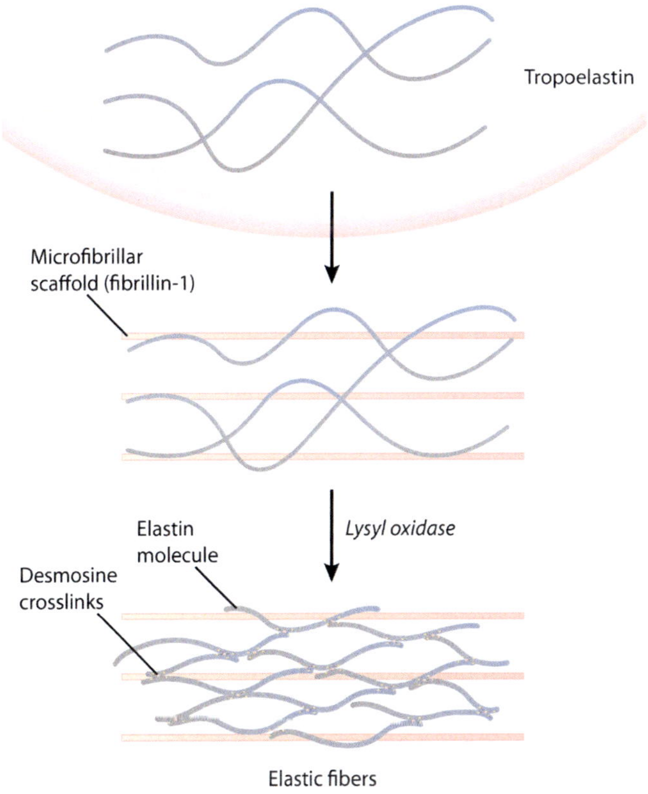

Figure 2.2.6 - Elastin synthesis

REVIEW QUESTIONS

1. A 71-year-old male is brought to the ED by his daughter due to tender gums and petechiae over the lower extremities. She states that he has lived alone for the past two years after his wife passed away. Since that time he has struggled with depression and finds little pleasure in eating. He states that he has mostly eaten meat, bread, and desserts. The physician on call suspects a nutrient deficiency resulting in impaired synthesis of an important molecule. What step in the synthesis of this molecule is most likely impaired?

- **Tender gums, petechiae, and a poor diet → scurvy**
- **The molecule described in the question is collagen**
- **Hydroxylation of the pro-α-chain requires vitamin C**
- **Deficiency of vitamin C → scurvy → ↓ hydroxylation of the pro-α-chain**

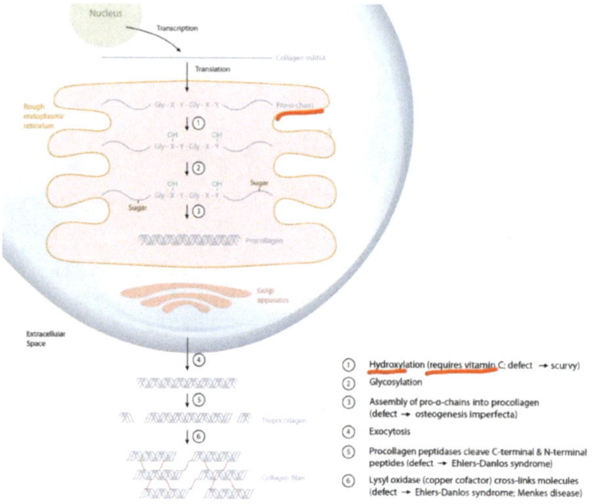

2. A 4-year-old boy is brought to the physician by his mother for a routine visit. While examining the patient the physician notices that he is able to extend his index finger backwards, allowing him to touch the posterior aspect of his wrist. Upon further questioning his mother states that he bruises easily. The physician suspects a genetic disorder resulting in impaired synthesis of an important molecule. What step in the synthesis of this molecule is most likely impaired?

- **Hypermobile joints and easy bruising → Ehlers-Danlos syndrome**
- **The molecule described in the question is collagen**
- **Ehlers-Danlos syndrome is caused by deficiencies of procollagen peptidase or lysyl oxidase**
- **Cleavage of procollagen terminals or formation of cross-links may be impaired**

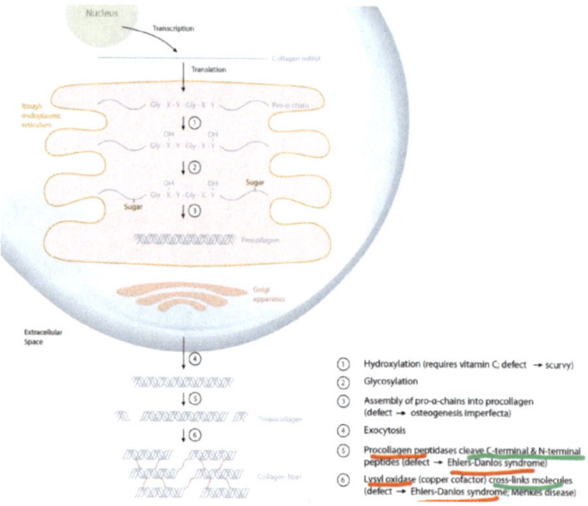

3. A 21-year-old male with no significant past medical history presents for a routine office visit. He is 6.5 feet tall and has long extremities. During cardiac auscultation of the left sternal border, a holosystolic murmur that radiates to the left axilla is heard. The physician suspects a genetic disorder resulting in a defective glycoprotein. What is the function of the glycoprotein most likely described above?

- **Marfanoid habitus, cardiac murmur, and defective glycoprotein (fibrillin-1) → Marfan syndrome**
- **Fibrillin-1 is a component of the microfibrils → scaffold for elastin**

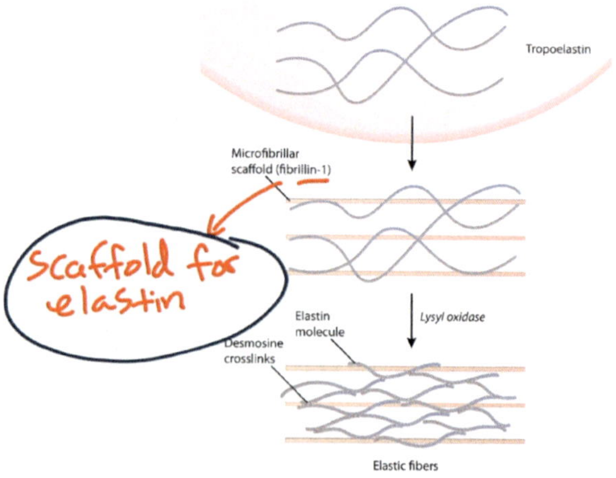

LABORATORY TECHNIQUES

Section I - PCR

I. Polymerase chain reaction (PCR) (Figure 2.3.1)

   A. A method of amplifying DNA

   B. Four elements are necessary for PCR

      1. A source DNA template
      2. Knowledge of the adjacent regions (flanking sequences) to the target that will be amplified (a DNA primer can then be utilized to bind to these regions)
      3. A DNA polymerase that can withstand high temperature (thermostable)
      4. Deoxynucleotide triphosphates

   C. There are three steps in the process of amplification

      1. Denaturing: this occurs by heating up the DNA template
      2. Annealing: the sample is cooled and primers adhere to the flanking regions of the target.
      3. Elongation: the sample is warmed and DNA polymerase copies the DNA

   D. The intensity of an amplified band on a gel can provide 'semi-quantitative' results.

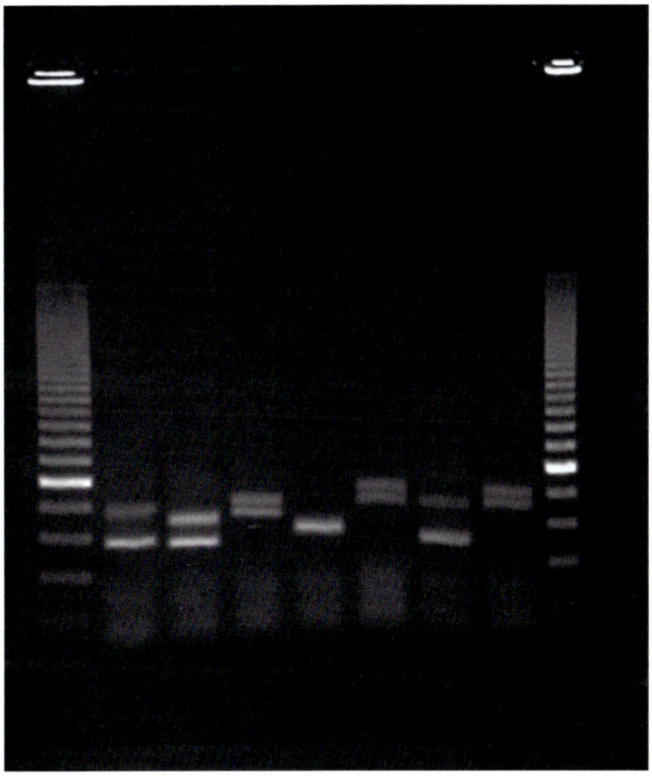

Figure 2.3.2 - DNA bands from electrophoresis

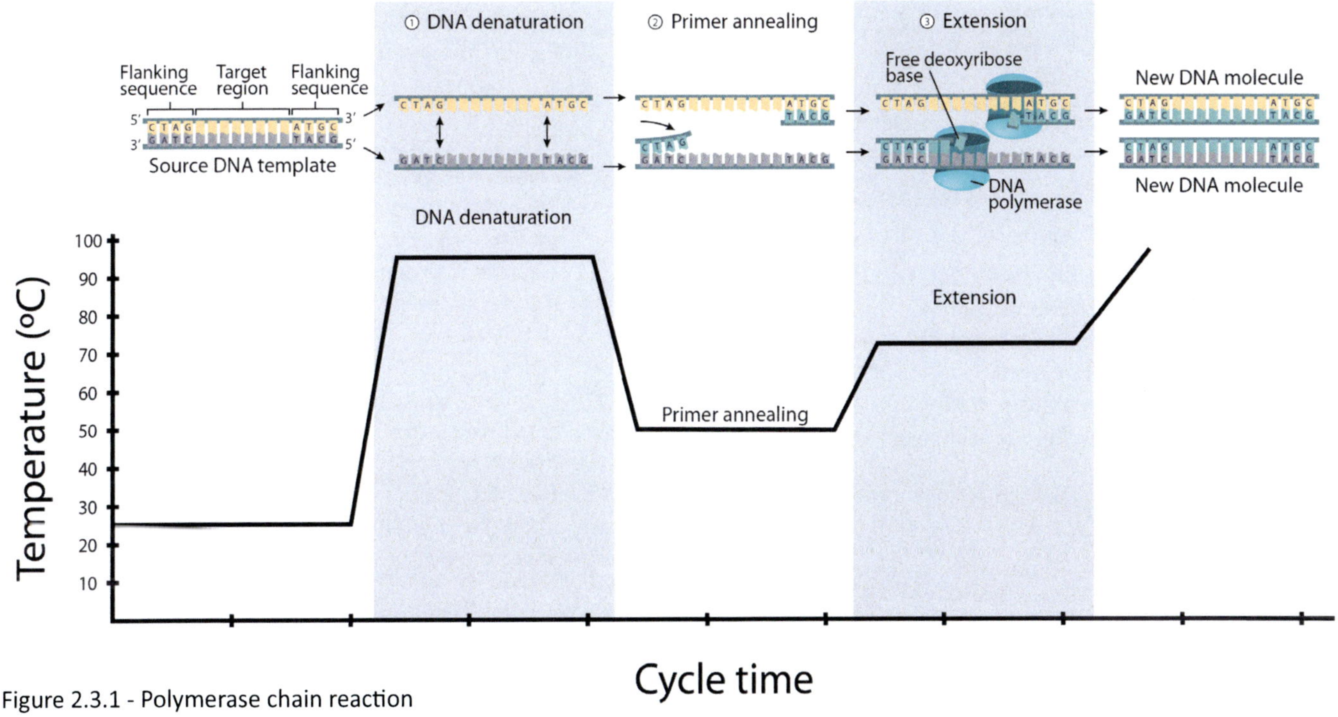

Figure 2.3.1 - Polymerase chain reaction

II. Real time PCR (Figure 2.3.3)

A. Single stranded DNA fluorescent used

B. As DNA polymerase replicates the DNA, the probe is removed and activated → light emitted

C. Fluorescence intensity reflects the quantity of DNA

D. Curve which crosses threshold line first had the highest concentration of DNA in the initial sample

III. Reverse transcription PCR

A. A template of cDNA is produced from a mRNA by reverse transcriptase.

B. The cDNA doesn't contain introns because it is made from mRNA.

C. This test is useful in measuring mRNA.

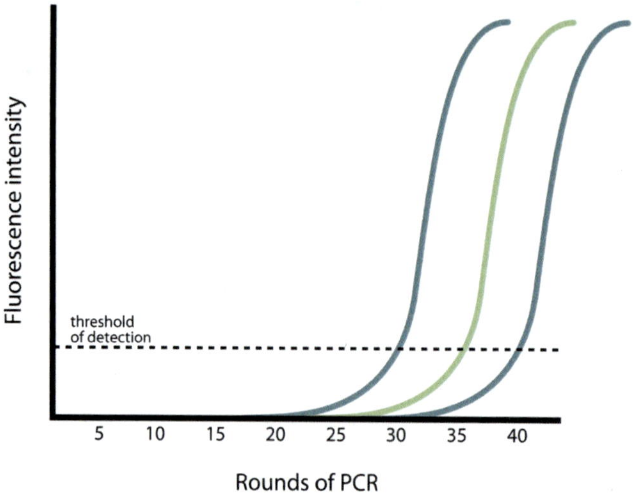

Figure 2.3.3 - Real time PCR

REVIEW QUESTIONS

1. A 37-year-old female has been working with an infertility specialist in an attempt to become pregnant. During *in vitro* fertilization, an egg is retrieved from the ovaries. The egg is then artificially inseminated and prepared for uterine implantation. However, the patient requests that the embryo be screened for genetic mutations prior to uterine implantation. A sample of DNA is obtained from the embryo and PCR is performed to screen for several genetic abnormalities including Huntington disease. A gene on chromosome 4 is amplified and the embryo produces a PCR product that is much larger than expected. What does the large PCR product most likely indicate about the embryo?

   - **Huntington disease → CAG trinucleotide repeat disorder on chromosome 4**
   - **Amplification of this region → product that was much larger than expected → patient must have CAG repeats resulting in a longer amplified region → embryo most likely has Huntington disease**

2. A 14-year-old boy is diagnosed with acute lymphoblastic leukemia. He is started on an aggressive chemotherapeutic regimen and receives regular follow up care. During one of these visits his treatment response is analyzed by using reverse transcription PCR. A bone marrow aspirate is obtained and mRNA created by a BCR/ABL translocation is then used as the template for real time PCR. How will the PCR product most likely differ from the BCR/ABL gene?

   - **BCR/ABL is usually associated with CML but can sometimes be associated with ALL**
   - **The mRNA produced by BCR/ABL represents malignancy and can be quantified to asses the treatment response**
   - **If the chemotherapeutic regimen is effective → ↓ mRNA**
   - **If the regimen is ineffective → ↑ mRNA**
   - **In order to quantify the mRNA it must be converted into cDNA to be amplified by real time PCR**
   - **The PCR product will lack introns (derived from mRNA) and the BCR/ABL gene will contain introns**

Section II - Blotting Procedures

I. Overview (Figure 2.3.4)

A. Southern blot: DNA

B. Northern blot: mRNA

C. Western blot: Proteins

D. Southwestern blot: DNA-binding proteins

E. Mnemonic: "SNoW DRoP"

II. Southern blot

A. DNA cleaved into small segments

B. Separated on a gel by electrophoresis

C. Transferred to a filter

D. Radiolabeled DNA probe added to the filter which binds to any complementary strands of DNA

E. DNA bound to the probe is visualized when the filter is exposed to film.

F. Restriction fragment length polymorphisms (i.e. sickle cell anemia)

III. Northern and western blot procedures are performed similarly to a southern blot procedure.

IV. Southwestern blot

A. Protein separated on a gel by electrophoresis

B. Transferred to a filter

C. Radiolabeled DNA probe added to the filter

D. If the DNA probe contains a protein binding region it will bind to the protein

E. The protein with an attached DNA probe will be visualized when the filter is exposed to the film

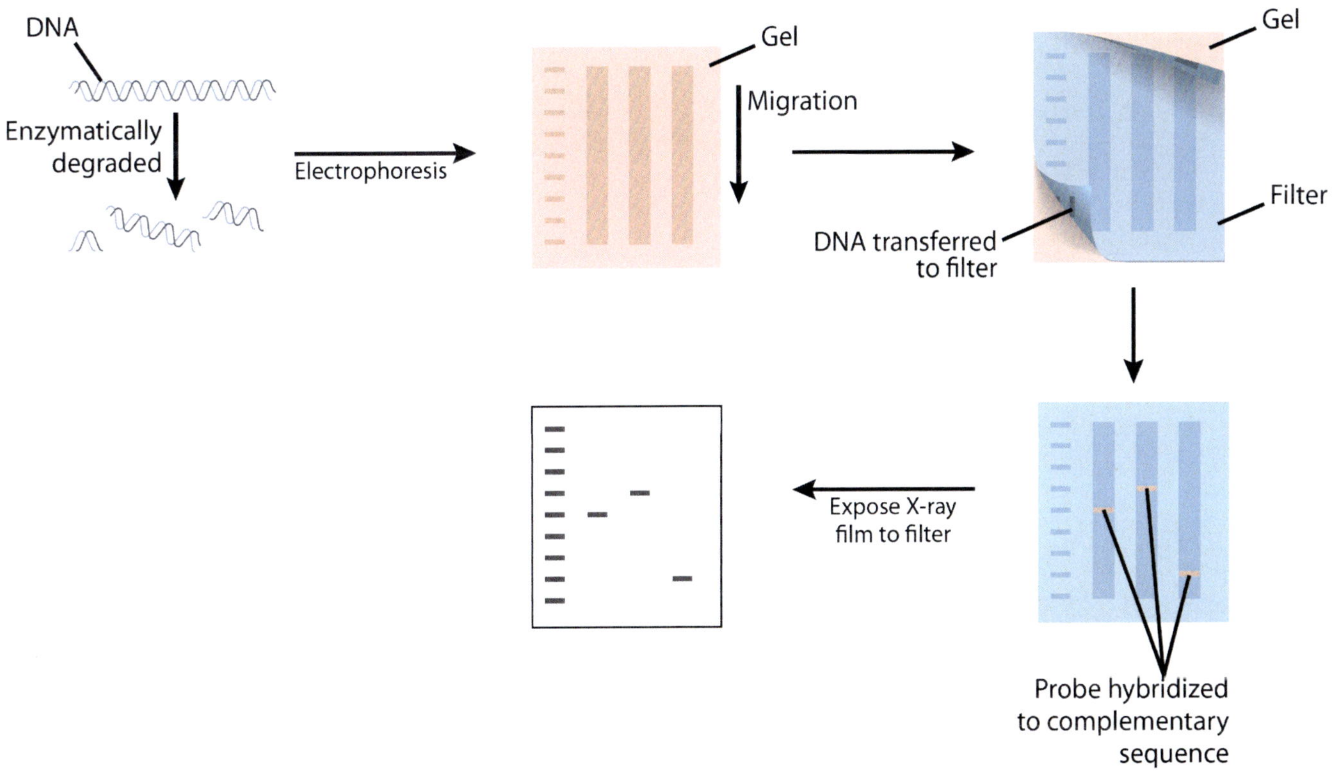

Figure 2.3.4 - Blotting procedures

REVIEW QUESTIONS

1. A pathologist is studying DNA replication from E. coli samples collected from patients with urinary tract infections. What blotting technique could be used to determine if a gene is being replicated?

    A) Northern blot
    B) Southern blot
    C) Western blot
    D) Southwestern blot

- **Southern blots are used to identify DNA**
- **DNA replication involves DNA so it could be best identified by using a southern blot (B)**

2. A newborn boy is brought to the physician for genetic testing. The father has familial adenomatous polyposis (FAP) and the mother is otherwise healthy. The patient's paternal grandfather also has FAP. DNA samples are obtained from the father, mother, paternal grandfather, maternal grandfather, and the patient. Southern blotting of restriction fragments from chromosome 5 near the APC gene are shown below.

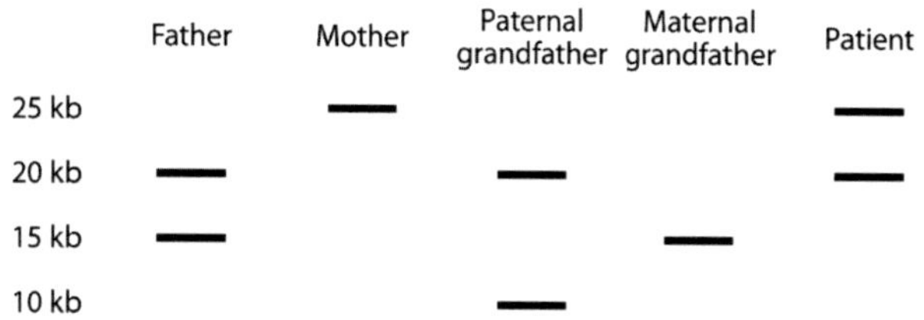

What can most likely be concluded about the findings shown above?

- **The father and paternal grandfather both have FAP (autosomal dominant condition that causes the colon to be covered in adenomatous polyps and progresses to cancer)**
- **The patient shares a restriction fragment with the father, paternal grandfather, and mother**
- **The mother is healthy → 25 kb fragment is normal**
- **The father and paternal grandfather have disease → 20 kb fragment is abnormal**
- **The patient most likely has FAP**

I. Overview

A. Method of analyzing cells (eg, cell markers, size, granularity).

B. A laser and a photodetector are used

C. Commonly used in conjunction with fluorescent labeled antibodies.

1. A fluorescent label is bound to an antibody.
2. The fluorescent-antibody complex is added to a solution of cells.
3. The solution is processed through a flow cytometer.

D. Clinical applications

1. Hematologic abnormalities (eg, lymphoma, leukemia, immunodeficiencies)

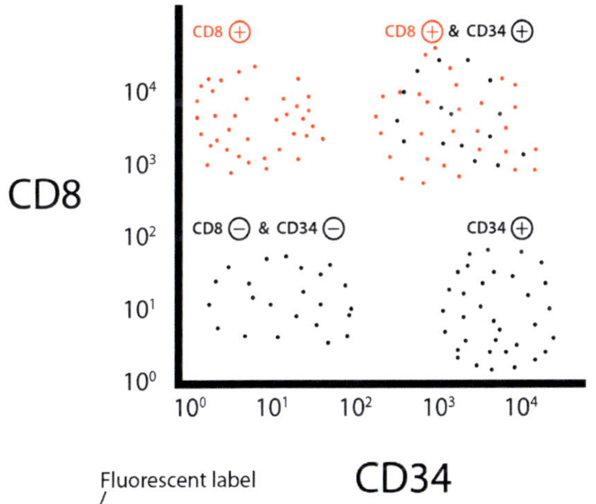

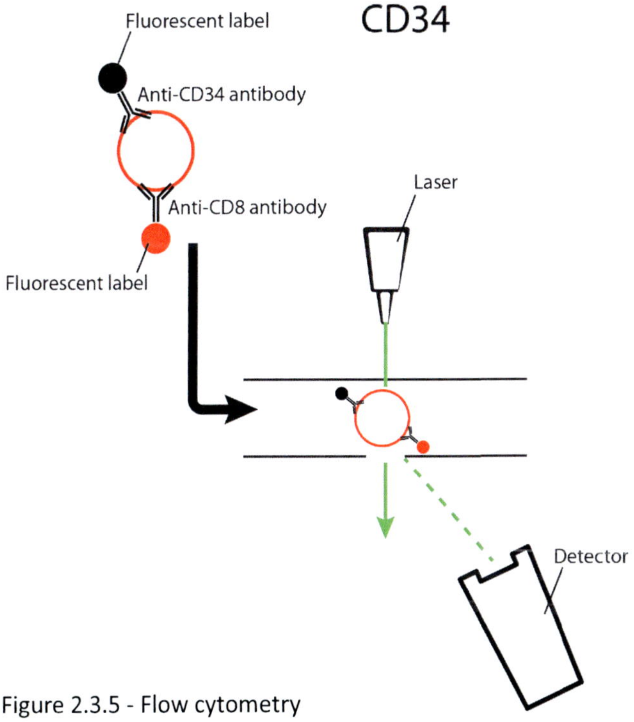

Figure 2.3.5 - Flow cytometry

REVIEW QUESTIONS

1. A 7-year-old girl presents with symptoms concerning for acute lymphoblastic leukemia (ALL). A sample of blood is obtained and sent to the lab for flow cytometry analysis. In T cell ALL, leukemic blasts are known to express CD2. A solution of fluorescent labeled anti-CD2 and anti-CD4 antibodies is mixed with the patient's blood and processed through a flow cytometry machine. The results are shown below.

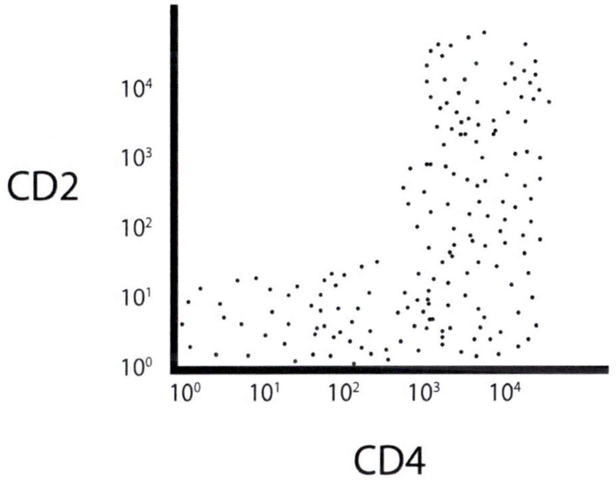

What can most likely be concluded based on the findings shown above?

- **The blast cells express the marker CD2**
- **The figure shows high concentrations of CD2 and CD4 in the top right quadrant → the results confirm the diagnosis of T cell ALL**

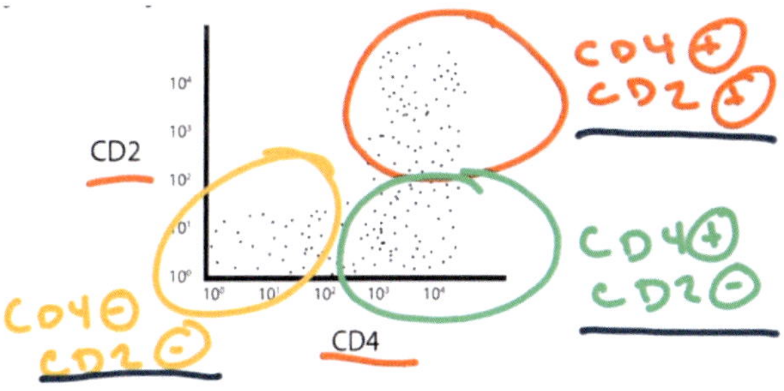

Section IV - Microarrays and ELISA

I. Microarrays (Figure 2.3.6)

   A. Consists of a plastic or silicon plate lined with probes (DNA sequences).

   B. A sample of cDNA that is labeled with fluorescent markers can be added to the plate.

   C. The sample cDNA that hybridizes to the complementary probe will fluoresce and can be analyzed by a computer.

   D. Commonly used to analyze gene expression.

II. ELISA

   A. Detects proteins in the blood (eg, antigens and antibodies).

   B. An enzyme is linked to an antibody.

   C. The enzyme-antibody complex produces a color change when substrate reacts with the enzyme.

   D. ELISA types include direct, indirect, sandwich, and competitive.

      1. Direct (the enzyme-antibody complex binds DIRECTLY to the antigen)

         a) Serum added to plate which coats the plate with antigens

         b) Plate is washed to remove the serum, but antigens remain bound to the plate

         c) Enzyme-antibody complex that is specific to the antigen of interest is added to the plate and then washed again

         d) Substrate specific for the enzyme is added to the plate

         e) Color change indicates positive ELISA

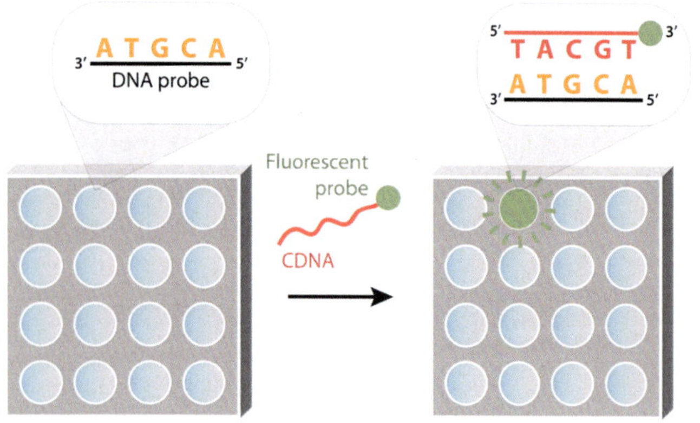

Figure 2.3.6 - Microarray

REVIEW QUESTIONS

1. A complication of myelodysplastic syndrome is the progression to acute myeloid leukemia (AML). Researchers have found that simultaneous expression of multiple gene mutations increases the risk of progression to AML. What laboratory technique would most likely be utilized in determining a patient's likelihood of progressing from myelodysplastic syndrome to AML?

   A) Southern blot
   B) ELISA
   C) Microarray
   D) Flow cytometry

   - **The question is describing gene expression → microarray would most likely be used (C)**

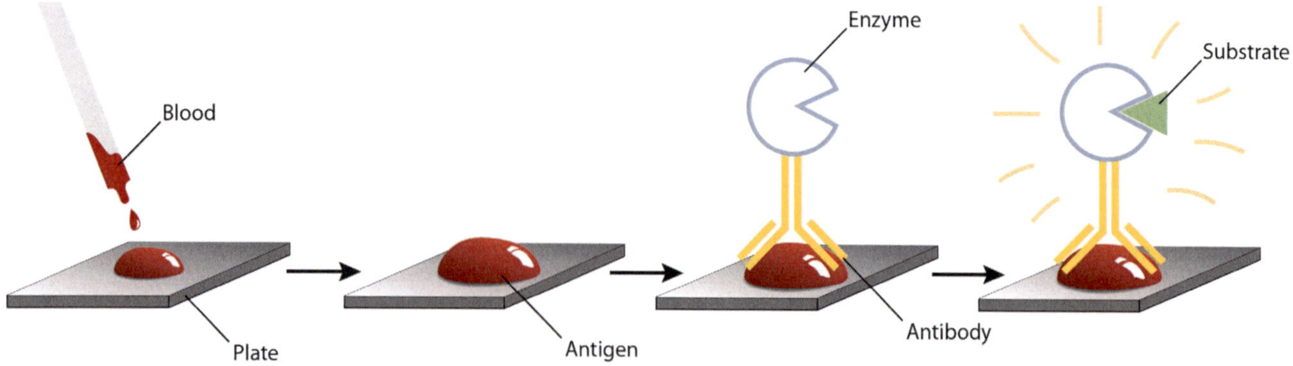

Figure 2.3.7 - Direct ELISA

Section V - Karyotyping and FISH

I. Karyotyping

A. Metaphase chromosomes are stained and placed in numerical order based upon size and morphology.

B. Commonly used to diagnose chromosomal abnormalities (eg, trisomy 21, Turner syndrome, etc.).

C. Often used in conjunction with fluorescence in situ hybridization (FISH).

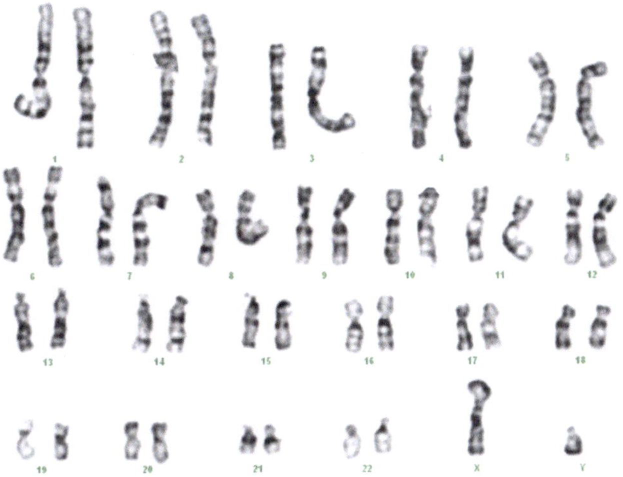

Figure 2.3.8 - Karyogram

II. FISH (Figures 2.3.9 and 2.3.10)

A. Fluorescent DNA/RNA probe binds to complementary region of interest on a chromosome which can then be visualized with fluorescence microscopy.

B. Visualized with fluorescence microscopy

C. Commonly used to identify gene and chromosomal abnormalities (duplications, translocations, and microdeletions).

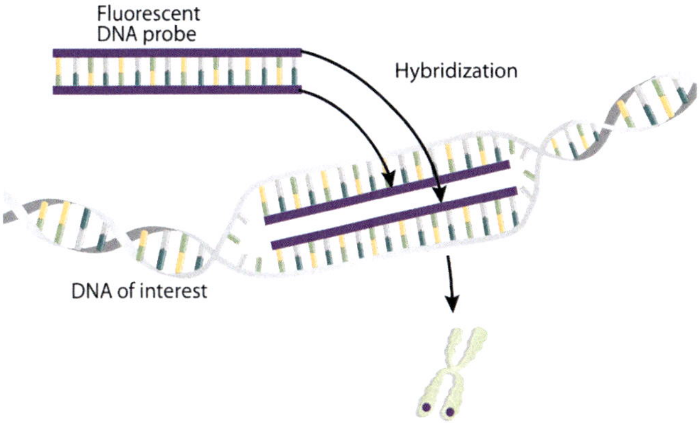

Figure 2.3.10 - FISH

REVIEW QUESTIONS

1. A 66-year-old male presents to with a 2-month history of fatigue, weight loss, night sweats, and several episodes of minor cuts causing excessive bleeding. A CBC reveals elevated WBCs. Laboratory analysis reveals decreased leukocyte alkaline phosphatase (LAP). A genetic abnormality is suspected. What laboratory technique will most likely be used to identify this patient's genetic abnormality?

   A) FISH
   B) Microarray
   C) ELISA
   D) Flow cytometry

- **The findings described are consistent with a hematologic malignancy (weight loss, night sweats, elevated WBCs, and decreased LAP)**
- **Decreased LAP is a unique finding in CML**
- **LAP is found in the secondary granules of granulocytes and is associated with inflammation**
- **Cells that fight infection → LAP positive**
- **Neoplastic cells → LAP negative**
- **CML results in a translocation of chromosomes 9 and 22 (t[9,22])**
- **Translocations can be identified using FISH (A)**

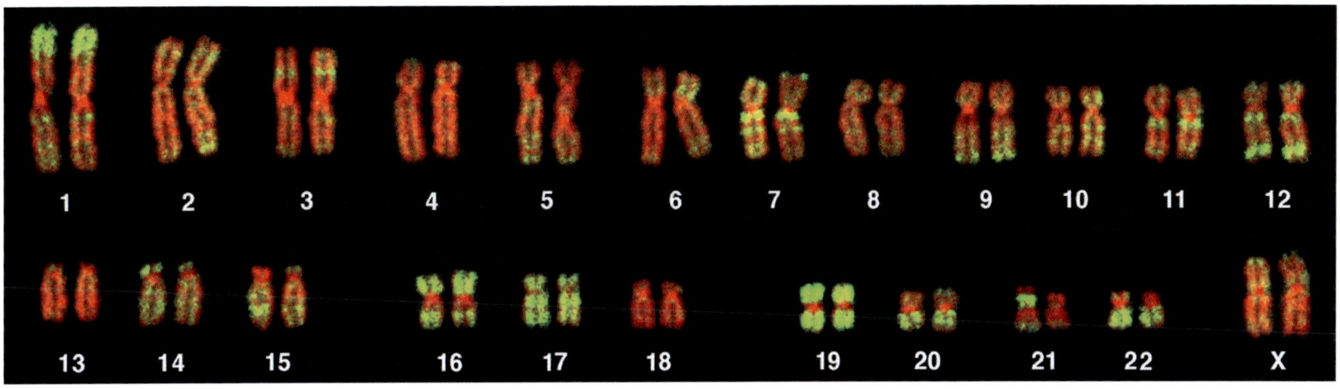

Figure 2.3.9 - FISH of a karyogram

Section VI - CRISPR/Cas9 & Molecular Cloning

I. CRISPR/Cas9 (Figure 2.3.11)

A. Bacteria-derived genome editing tool.

B. Cas9 is an endonuclease that unzips and cleaves dsDNA.

C. A guide RNA (gRNA) directs the Cas9 enzyme to a complementary DNA target sequence and a cut is made.

D. Gap region is repaired through nonhomologous end joining (error prone) or a genetically engineered sequence of DNA (decreases risk of errors).

II. Molecular cloning (Figure 2.3.12)

A. Eukaryotic mRNA is reverse transcribed into cDNA.

B. The cDNA is inserted into a plasmid containing an antibiotic resistant gene.

C. Recombinant plasmid is inserted into bacteria (transformation).

D. Sample is cultured on a medium containing antibiotics.

E. Bacteria that successfully absorbed the plasmid will survive, and those that did not properly absorb the plasmid will die.

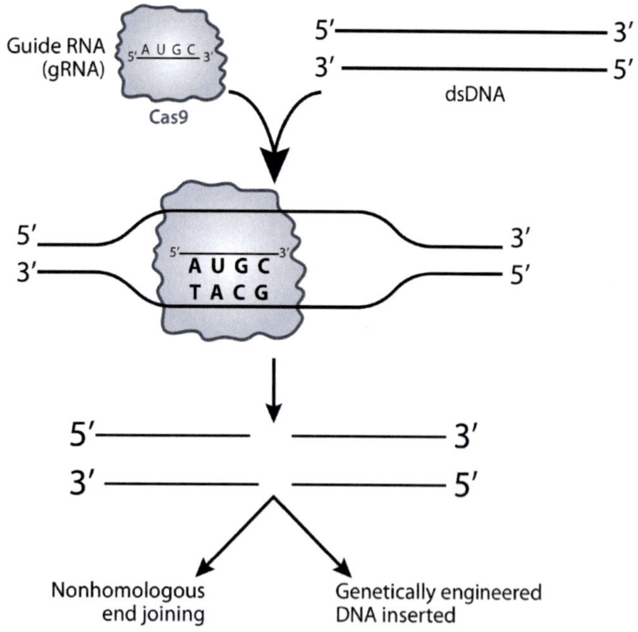

Figure 2.3.11 - CRISPR/Cas9

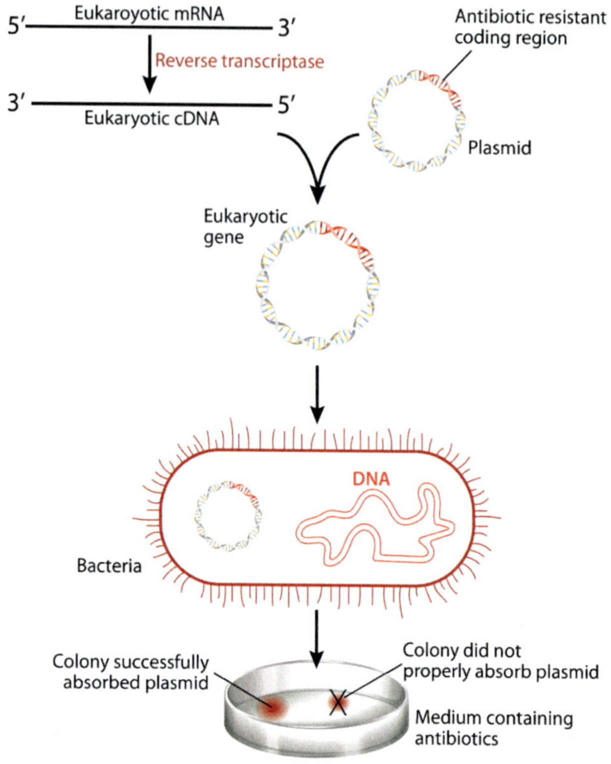

Figure 2.3.12 - Molecular cloning

REVIEW QUESTIONS

1. A pharmaceutical company is attempting to synthesize insulin for use as a commercialized medication. What lab technique would most likely be used to achieve this goal?

- **Molecular cloning**
- **Synthetically derived human insulin is synthesized by bacteria in a lab, purified, and then used as a medication for diabetic patients**

GENETICS

Section I - Genetics Overview

Term	Definition	Example
Codominance	Multiple alleles associated with a gene are simultaneously expressed	Blood groups
Incomplete penetrance	Individuals who carry the mutant genotype but do not express the mutant phenotype	BRCA1 may cause breast cancer in one individual but the other individual may remain cancer free
Variable expressivity	Variability in the phenotype expressed by individuals with the same genotype	Patients with neurofibromatosis type I (NF1) may have cutaneous neurofibromas covering the entire body or only a small part of the body (all patients have 100% penetrance) (Figure 2.4.2)
Pleiotropy	One gene is responsible for multiple phenotypic manifestations	Homocystinuria causes multiple symptoms affecting multiple organs (lens dislocation, DVTs, Marfanoid habitus, and intellectual disability)
Anticipation	The tendency of a disease to occur earlier or to be more severe in succeeding generations	Huntington disease
Loss of heterozygosity	Refers to the idea that tumor suppressor genes must develop mutations in both alleles before cancer will develop	Retinoblastoma (Figure 2.4.3)
Germline mosaicism	The presence of multiple, genetically distinct cell lines in the gametes	(Figure 2.4.4)
Somatic mosaicism	The presence of multiple, genetically distinct cell lines within the cells that form the body	Turner syndrome McCune-Albright syndrome (Figure 2.4.5)
Locus heterogeneity	The same phenotype can be caused by mutations at different loci	Albinism
Allelic heterogeneity	The same phenotype can be caused by mutations in the same locus	β-thalassemia
Heteroplasmy	The presence of both mutated and normal mitochondrial genomes within a single cell	Mitochondrial disorders (Figure 2.4.6)
Dominant negative mutation	The mutation results in a dominant effect	A nonfunctional protein prevents another normal protein from functioning properly

Table 2.4.1 - Genetic terms

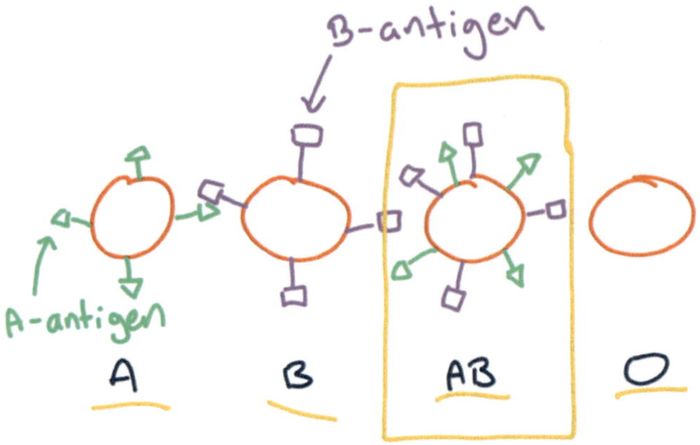

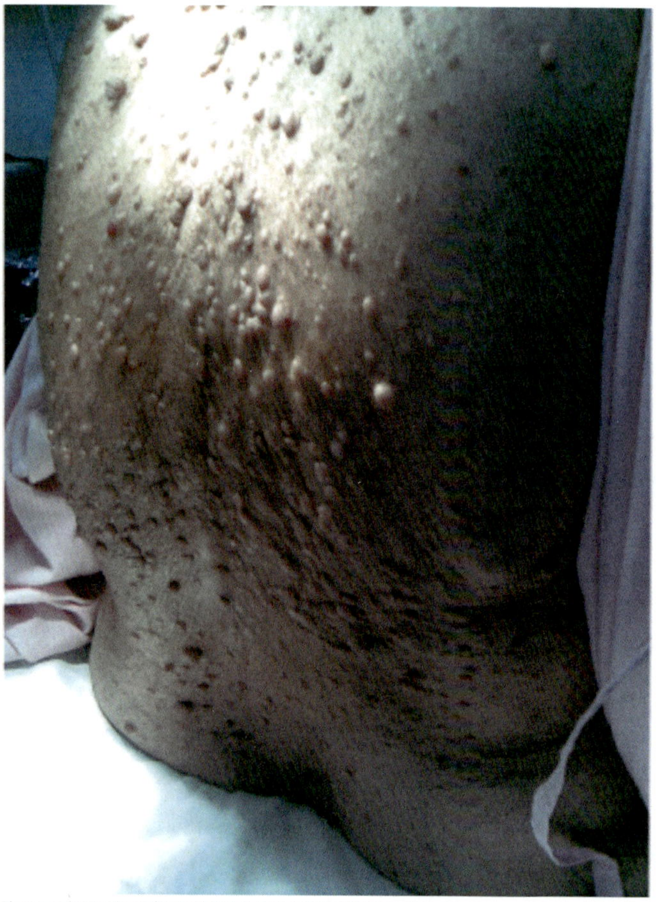

Photo Credit: By Almazi (Author) [Public domain], via Wikimedia Commons

Figure 2.4.1 - Neurofibromas

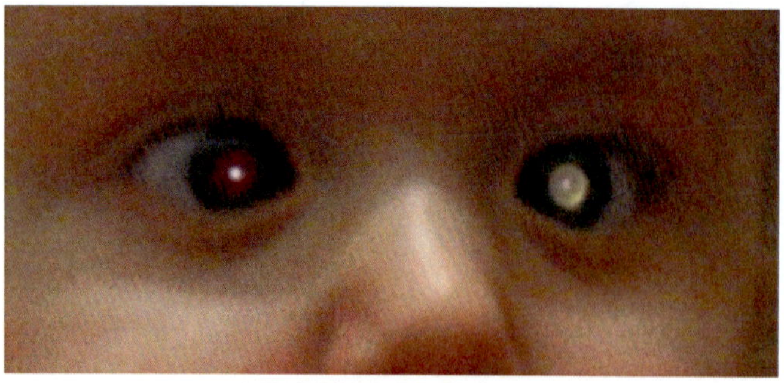

By J Morley-Smith [Public domain], from Wikimedia Commons

Photo Credit: By J Morley-Smith [Public domain], from Wikimedia Commons

Figure 2.4.2 - Retinoblastoma

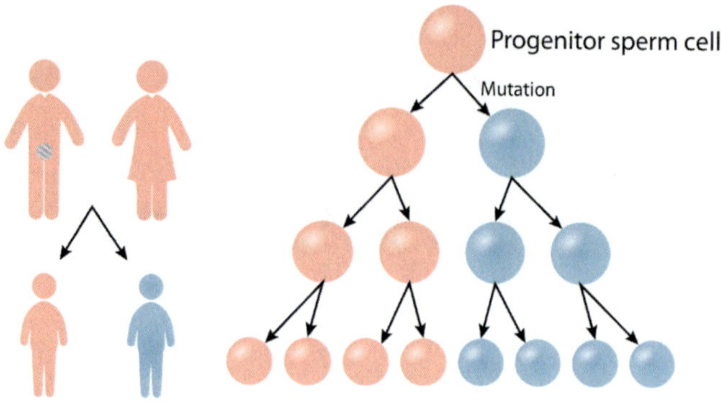

Figure 2.4.3 - Germline mosaicism

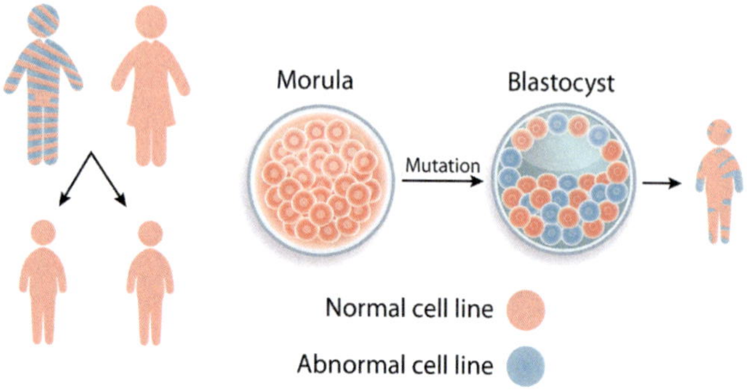

Figure 2.4.4 - Somatic mosaicism

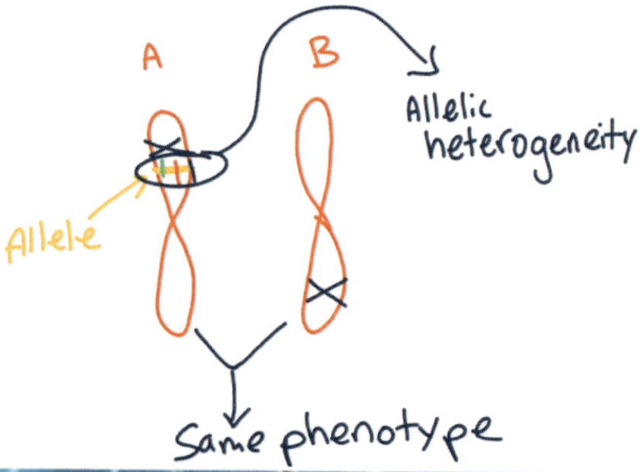

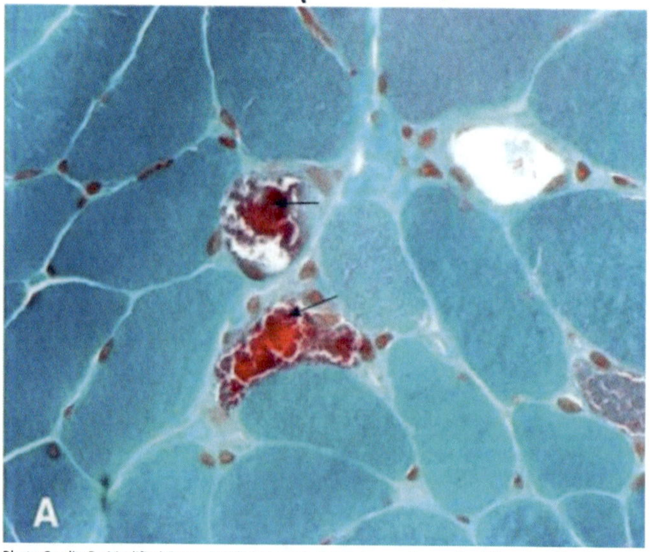

Photo Credit: By Modified Gomori trichrome stain showing several ragged red fibers.jpg: Abu-Amero KK, Al-Dhalaan H, Bohlega S, Hellani A, Taylor RW.derivative work: CopperKettle [CC BY 2.0 (https://creativecommons.org/licenses/by/2.0)], via Wikimedia Commons

Figure 2.4.5 - Gomori trichrome stain of ragged-appearing muscle fibers

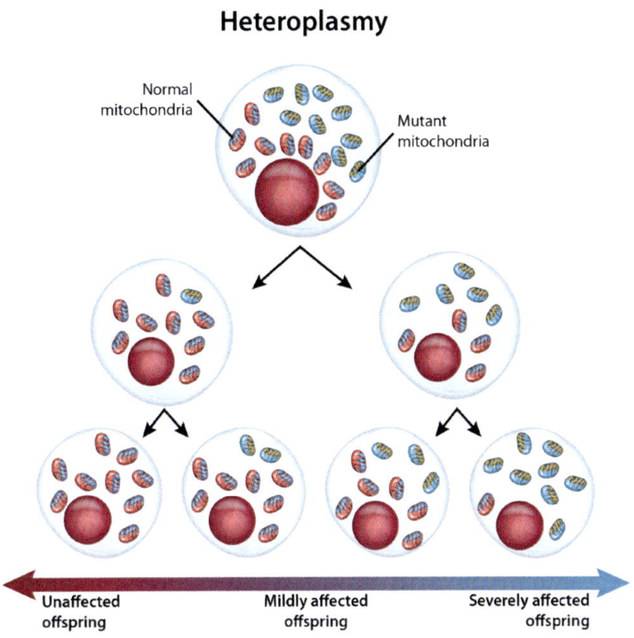

Figure 2.4.6 - Heteroplasmy

REVIEW QUESTIONS

1. A 1-day-old boy is born to a healthy 25-year-old female at term. On exam the boy is noted to have upslanting palpebral fissures, a single palmar crease bilaterally, and prominent epicanthal folds. FISH analysis on cultured fibroblasts shows that 70% of the cells have 47 chromosomes while 30% of the cells have 46 chromosomes. What genetic principle most likely explains these findings?
    - A) Meiotic nondisjunction
    - B) Germline mosaicism
    - C) Somatic mosaicism
    - D) Loss of heterozygosity
    - E) Variable expressivity

- **Correct answer is C**
- **Upslanting palpebral fissures, a single palmar crease bilaterally, and prominent epicanthal folds → Down syndrome**
- **FISH reveals two distinct cell lines (70% of the cells have 47 chromosomes while 30% have 46 chromosomes) → somatic mosaicism**

REVIEW QUESTIONS

2. A 41-year-old female presents to the physician for chronic muscle weakness. A skeletal muscle biopsy reveals ragged-appearing muscle fibers. DNA analysis reveals a mutation in 70% of the mitochondrial DNA. The physician is concerned about the possibility of the disease affecting the patient's children. However, the patient states that none of her children have any symptoms. What genetic principle most likely explains the absence of symptoms in this patient's children?

- **Heteroplasmy**
- **The patient has chronic muscle weakness and a mutation in 70% of her mitochondrial DNA yet none of her children have symptoms**
- **The 30% of her normal mitochondria can be passed onto her children resulting in unaffected offspring**
- **Mitochondrial diseases usually present with muscle weakness and a biopsy will reveal ragged-appearing muscle fibers**

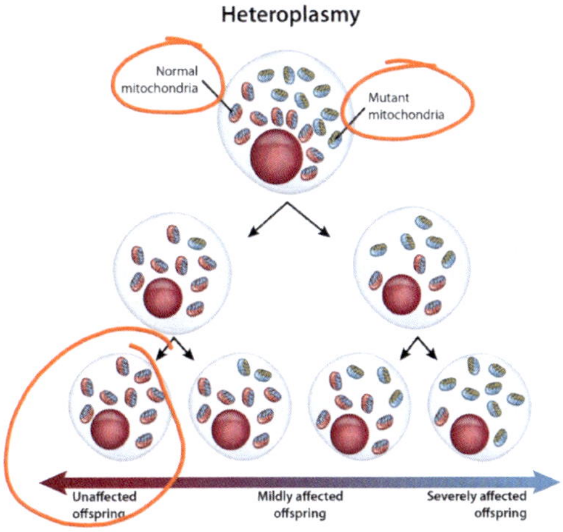

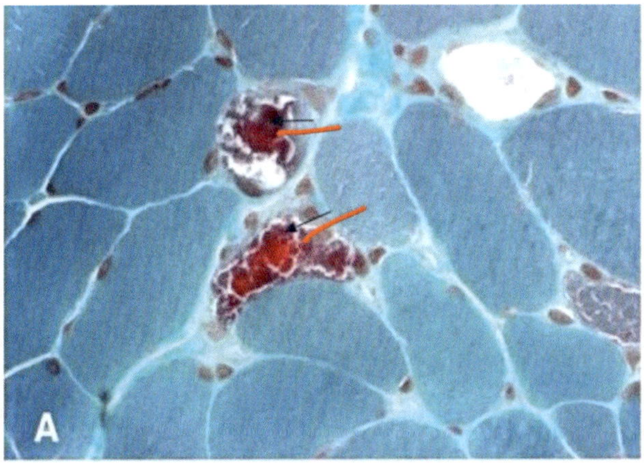

Section II - Imprinting and Uniparental Disomy

I. Imprinting

A. An offspring's gene expression becomes parent-specific due to inactivation of the opposite parent's allele.

B. DNA methylation suppresses transcription resulting in alterations in gene expression.

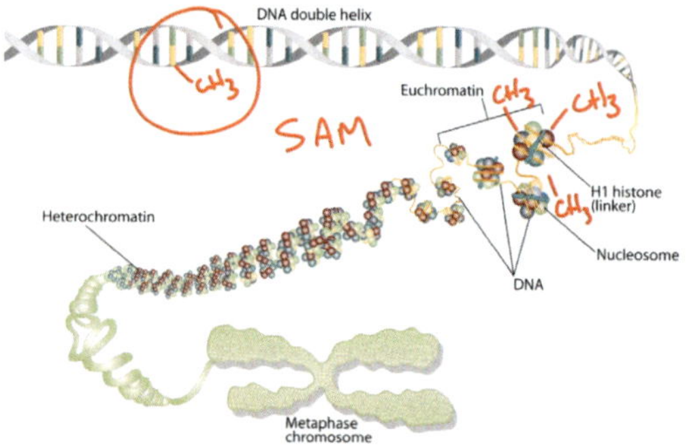

II. Prader-Willi syndrome (Figure 2.4.7)

A. The maternal region of 15q11-q13 which contains the PWS gene is normally silenced.

B. The paternal region contains an active version of the PWS gene.

C. A deletion or mutation of the paternal PWS gene results in Prader-Willi syndrome.

D. Symptoms include obesity, hyperphagia, intellectual disability, hypogonadism, hypotonia, and temperature instability.

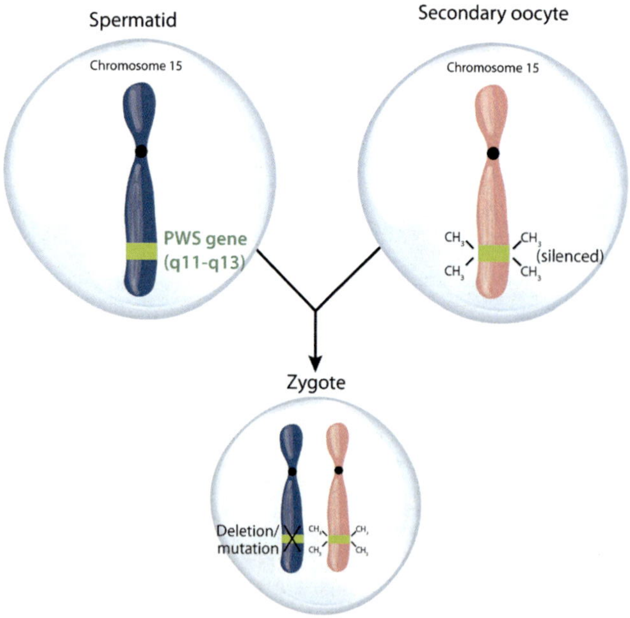

Figure 2.4.7 - Prader-Willi syndrome

III. Angelman syndrome (Figure 2.4.8)

A. The paternal region of 15q11-q13 which contains the UBE3A gene is normally silenced.

B. The maternal region contains an active version of the UBE3A gene.

C. A deletion or mutation of the maternal UBE3A gene results in Angelman syndrome.

D. Symptoms include inappropriate laughter, intellectual disability, seizures, and ataxia.

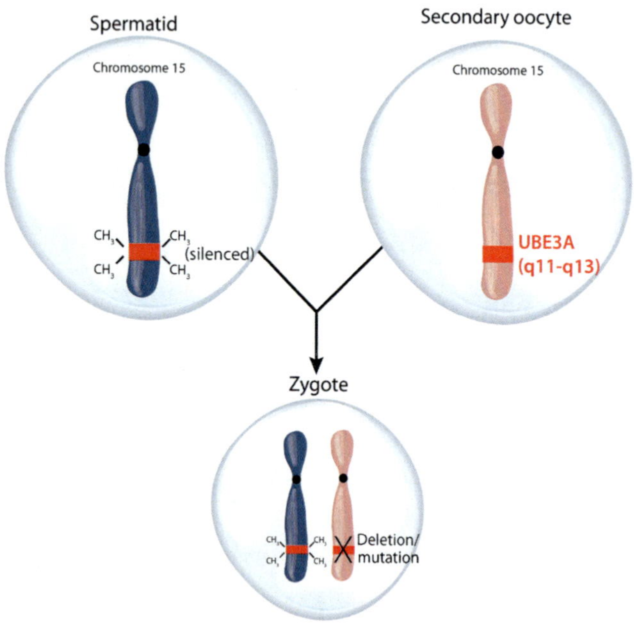

Figure 2.4.8 - Angelman syndrome

IV. Uniparental disomy (Figures 2.4.9 and 2.4.10)

A. Can cause Angelman syndrome and Prader-Willi syndrome

B. Two copies of a chromosome are inherited from one parent and no copies are inherited from the other parent

C. Caused by nondisjunction followed by the loss of genetic information

D. Meiosis I nondisjunction → heterodisomy

E. Meiosis II nondisjunction → isodisomy

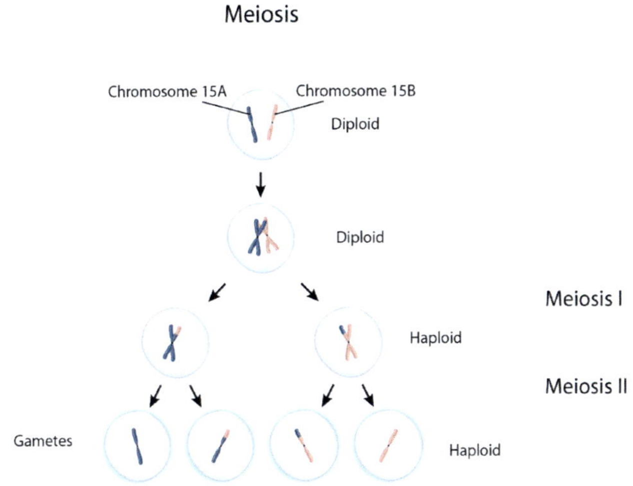

Figure 2.4.9 - Meiosis

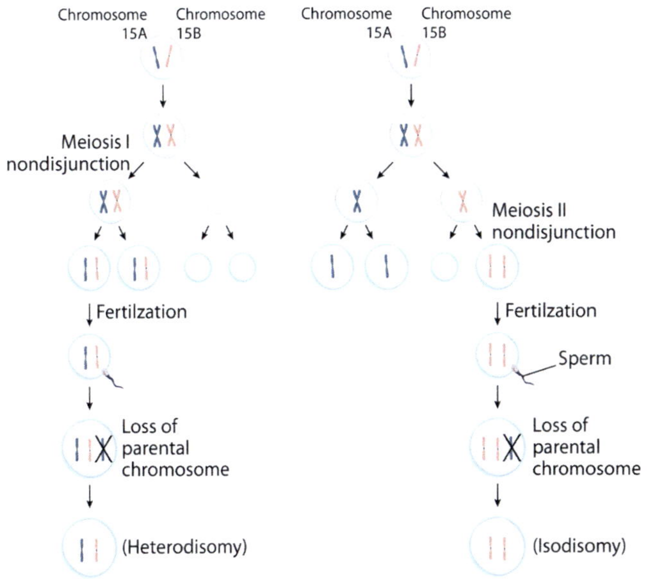

Figure 2.4.10 - Uniparental disomy

REVIEW QUESTIONS

1. A 5-year-old boy is found to have hyperphagia, obesity, and intellectual disability. Cytogenetic analysis reveals a deletion involving chromosome 15q11-q13. Which of the following is most likely true of this patient?

   A) The maternally inherited chromosome 15q11-q13 contains a deletion
   B) The paternally inherited chromosome 15q11-q13 is methylated
   C) The paternally inherited chromosome 15q11-q13 contains a deletion
   D) The maternally inherited chromosome 15q11-q13 is acetylated

- **Correct answer is C**
- **Hyperphagia, obesity, intellectual disability, and a deletion of chromosome 15q11-q13 → Prader-Willi syndrome**
- **Caused by a deletion/mutation of the paternal region of chromosome 15q11-q13**

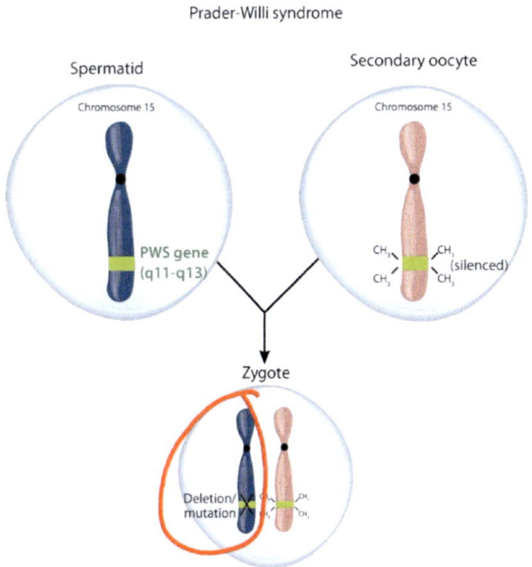

REVIEW QUESTIONS

2. A 3-year-old boy is found to have obesity, hyperphagia, and intellectual disability. Restriction fragment length polymorphism (RFLP) analysis is performed to determine the origin of the patient's genetic defect. DNA samples are obtained and exposed to a restriction enzyme. Southern blotting of restriction fragments from chromosome 15 are shown below.

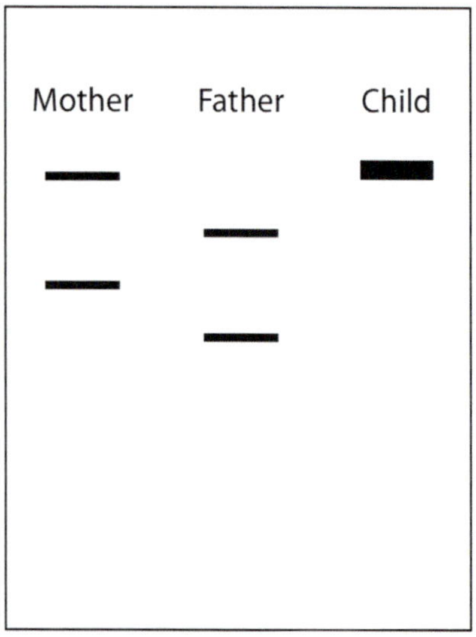

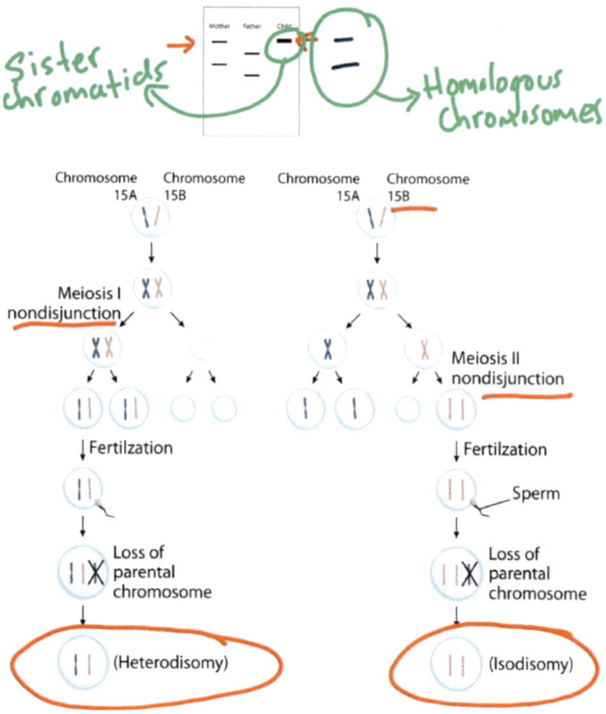

What can most likely be concluded about the findings shown above?

A) The boy inherited two copies of chromosome 15 from his mother due to nondisjunction of meiosis I
B) The boy inherited two copies of chromosome 15 from his mother due to nondisjunction of meiosis II
C) The boy inherited one heavily methylated copy of chromosome 15 from his mother
D) The boy inherited one heavily acetylated copy of chromosome 15 from his mother

- **Answer is B**
- **Obesity, hyperphagia, and intellectual disability → Prader-Willi syndrome**
- **RFLP from chromosome 15 are represented by the bands in the image above**
- **The child's band lines up with the band of the mother but is twice as thick → inheritance of two identical sister chromatids (they are identical so they produce equal size restriction fragments) → nondisjunction of meiosis II**

Section III - Linkage Disequilibrium

I. Independent assortment (Figure 2.4.11)

A. Chromosomes segregate independently of one another during meiosis.

B. Alleles that are located on separate chromosomes get sorted into gametes independently of one another.

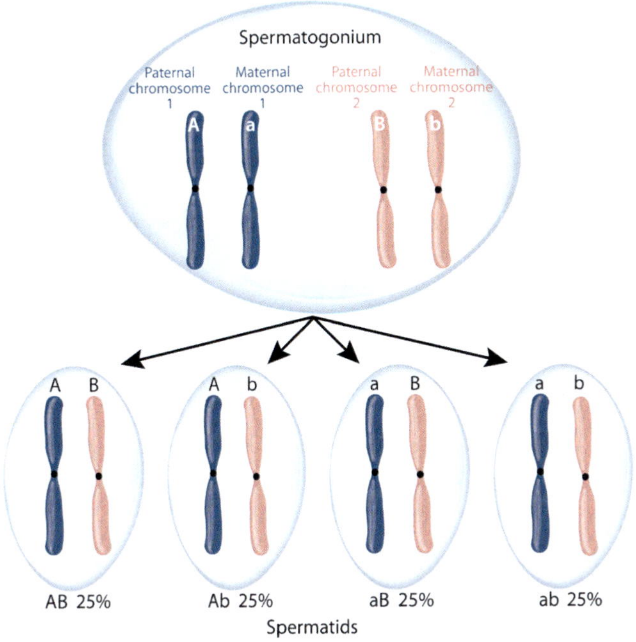

Figure 2.4.11 - Independent assortment

II. Linkage equilibrium (Figure 2.4.12)

A. Linkage: two alleles are located on the same chromosome.

B. Linkage equilibrium: the frequency of alleles inherited from one parent in a given population have the same value that they would have if the alleles at each locus were combined at random.

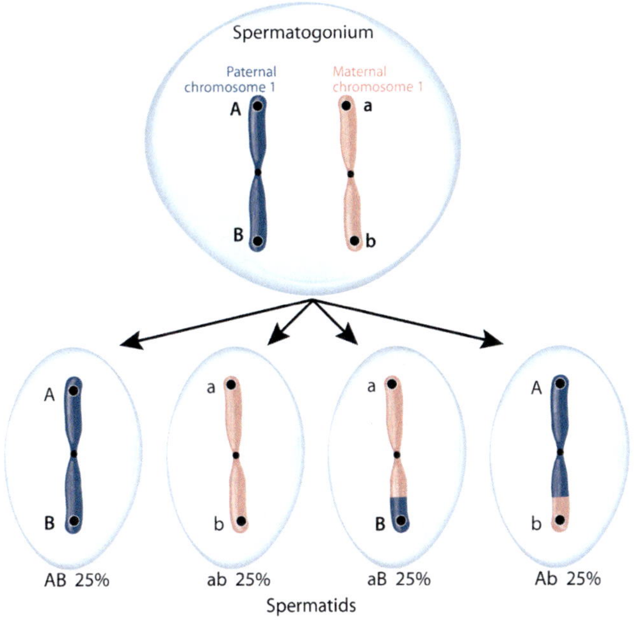

Figure 2.4.12 - Linkage equilibrium

III. Linkage disequilibrium

A. Tendency of alleles to be transmitted together more or less often than expected by chance alone.

B. Usually caused by close proximity of genes on the same chromosome.

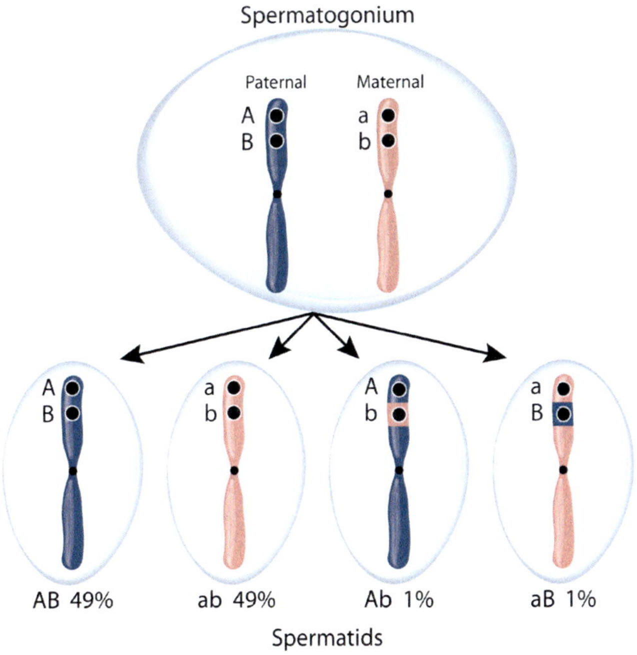

Figure 2.4.13 - Linkage disequilibrium

REVIEW QUESTIONS

1. Two regions on the same chromosome are sequenced using PCR. The frequency of the corresponding alleles are then analyzed in a population. The frequency of allele A is found to be 0.5 and the frequency of allele B is 0.5. Assuming normal linkage equilibrium, what is the expected frequency of AB?

- **0.25**
- **Allele A occurs 50% of the time and allele B occurs the other 50% of the time**
- **If the two alleles are in linkage equilibrium then the probability of them being inherited together is 0.25 (0.5 x 0.5 = 0.25)**
- **Linkage equilibrium refers to alleles that are on the SAME chromosome**
- **During meiosis, segments of the chromosomes break and are transferred to the homologous chromosome (even if two alleles are on the same chromosome, they may not always be inherited together)**
- **Two alleles on the same chromosome that are far apart from one another behave as if they were on separate chromosomes (↑ distance → ↑ likelihood of recombination to occur → linkage equilibrium [there is an equal probability of inheriting each allele just as if each allele were on a different chromosome])**

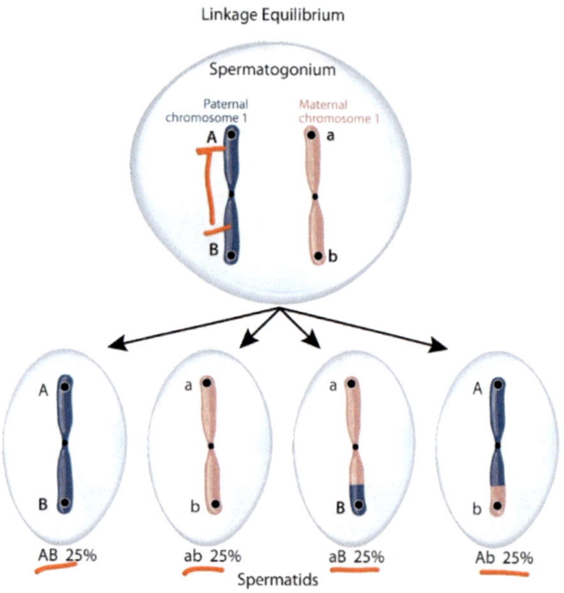

2. Two regions on the same chromosome are sequenced using PCR. The frequency of the corresponding alleles are then analyzed in a population. The frequency of allele A is found to be 0.5 and the frequency of allele B is 0.5. However, the frequency of AB is found to be 0.49 in the same population. What genetic principle most likely explains these findings?

- **Linkage disequilibrium**
- **Two alleles on the same chromosome with frequencies of 0.5 and 0.5 should result in a combined frequency of 0.25 (assuming normal linkage equilibrium)**
- **However, in the stem we're told that the frequency of AB is 0.49 (much higher than expected)**
- **If two alleles on the same chromosome are physically close together then there is a decreased probability that recombination will occur at this region (there are fewer places where the chromosomes can break so recombination only occurs a small percentage of the time) → linkage disequilibrium**

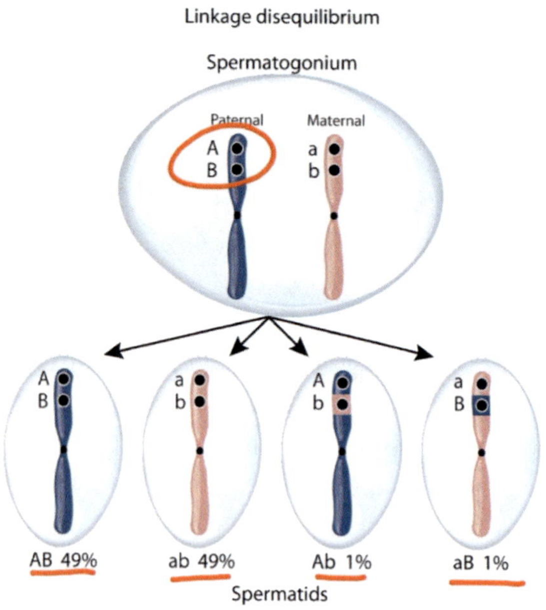

Section IV - Pedigrees

I. Pedigree (Figure 2.4.14)

   A. A diagram representing the occurrence of an inherited trait from one generation to the next.

   B. Unaffected individual → white box

   C. Affected individual → colored box

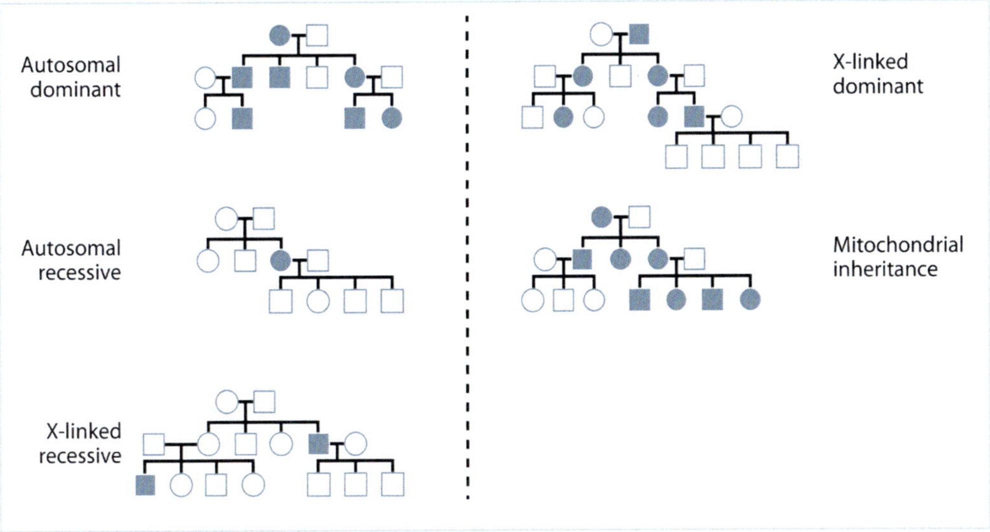

Figure 2.4.14 - Pedigree overview

II. Autosomal dominant inheritance (Figure 2.4.15)

   A. Individuals that exhibit the trait will have the genotype “AA” or “Aa”

   B. Tends to affect both males and females in each generation

   C. Will exhibit male-to-male transmission

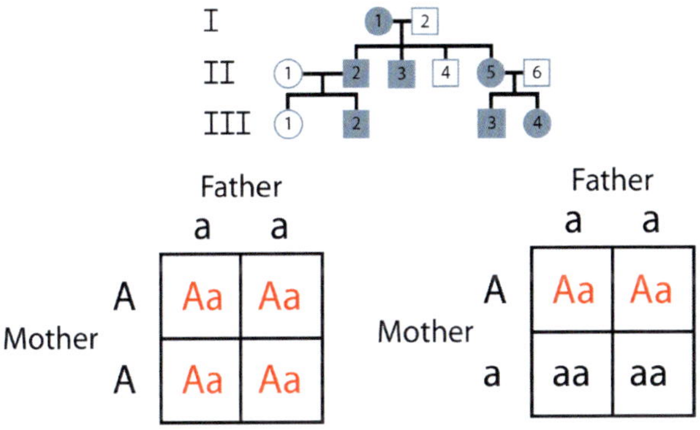

Figure 2.4.15 - Autosomal dominant pedigree

III. Autosomal recessive inheritance (Figure 2.4.16)

   A. Individuals affected will have the genotype “aa”

   B. Tends to skip generations

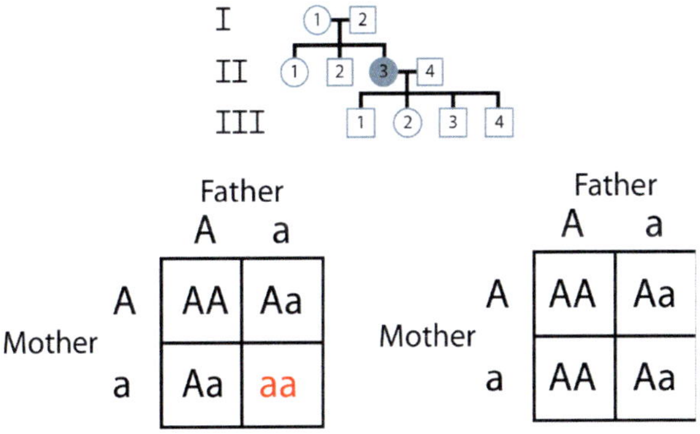

Figure 2.4.16 - Autosomal recessive pedigree

IV. X-linked recessive inheritance (Figure 2.4.17)

   A. Males are generally the only ones affected

   B. No male-to-male transmission

   C. Skewed lyonization can result in an affected female

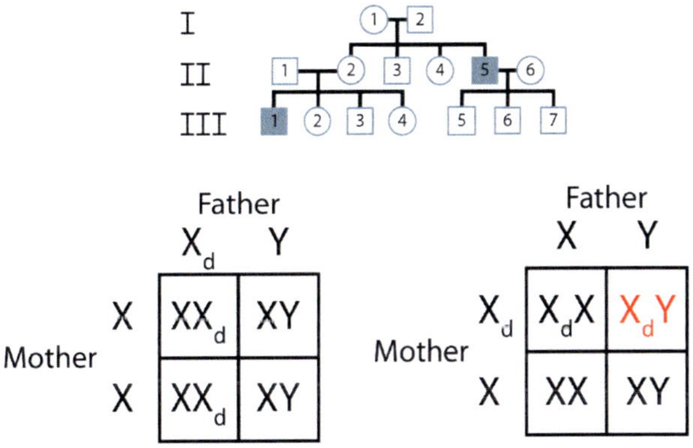

Figure 2.4.17 - X-linked recessive pedigree

V. X-linked dominant inheritance (Figure 2.4.18)

   A. Males and females are affected

   B. No male-to-male transmission

VI. Mitochondrial inheritance (Figure 2.4.19)

   A. Only transmitted through the mother because the mitochondria in sperm do not enter the ovum during fertilization

   B. Mitochondrial diseases exhibit heteroplasmy

   C. Findings include muscle tissue damage with a biopsy revealing “ragged-appearing muscle fibers”

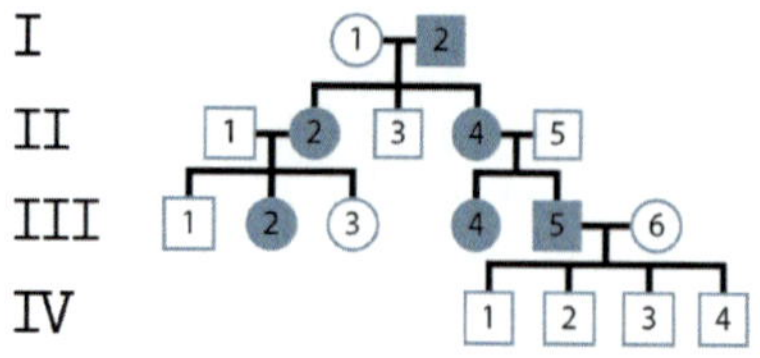

		Father X	Father Y
Mother	X_D	X_DX	X_DY
	X	XX	XY

		Father X_D	Father Y
Mother	X	XX_D	XY
	X	XX_D	XY

Figure 2.4.18 - X-linked dominant pedigree

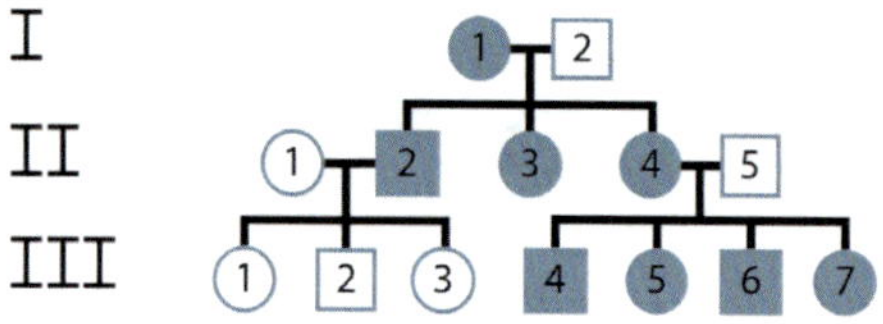

Figure 2.4.19 - Mitochondrial pedigree

REVIEW QUESTIONS

1. Based on the pedigree below, what can most likely be concluded about the genotype of I, 1?

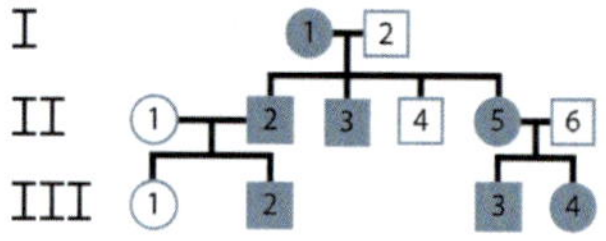

		Father a	Father a
Mother	A	Aa	Aa
	A	Aa	Aa

		Father a	Father a
Mother	A	Aa	Aa
	a	aa	aa

- **She is heterozygous (Aa)**
- **Males and females affected across multiple generations with male-to-male transmission → autosomal dominant inheritance**
- **The father indicated by I,2 must be homozygous recessive (aa) because he does not express the trait**
- **The mother indicated by I,1 must be heterozygous (Aa) because one of her offspring indicated by II,4 does not express the trait (aa).**
- **A genotype of AA would have resulted in all of her children expressing the trait which is not the case**

REVIEW QUESTIONS

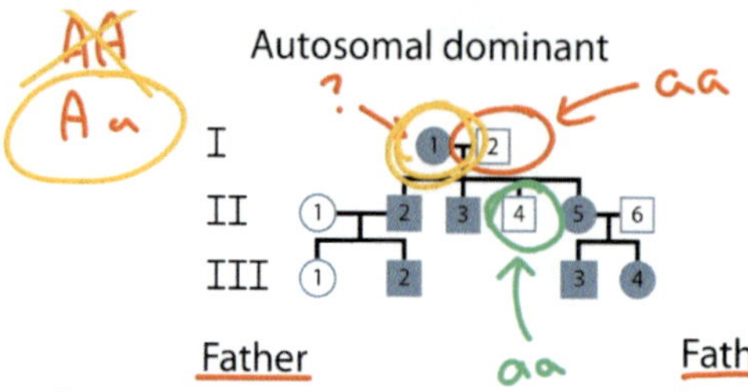

		Father a	Father a
Mother	A	Aa	Aa
	A	Aa	Aa

		Father a	Father a
Mother	A	Aa	Aa
	a	aa	aa

2. A 25-year-old male is brought to the physician for a routine visit. He has a genetic condition affecting multiple family members. The pedigree is shown below. The patient is shown at III, 5.

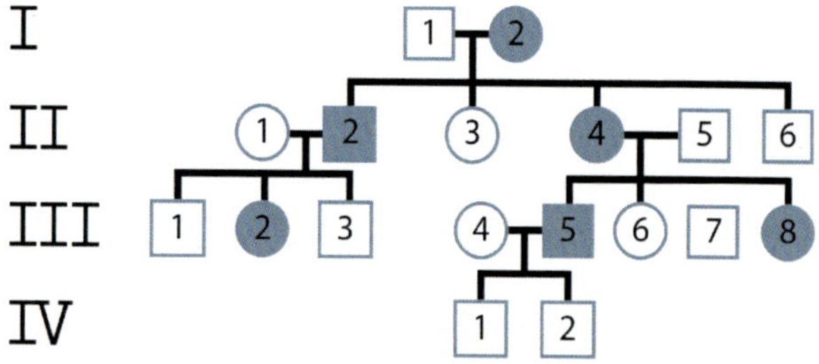

Based on these findings, what can most likely be concluded about this man's condition?

A) He has a fibroblast growth factor receptor 3 (FGFR3) mutation
B) His colon is covered with adenomatous polyps
C) He has autism, large ears, and macroorchidism
D) He has muscle weakness caused by a frameshift mutation

- **Correct answer is C**
- **Multiple generations are affected but there is no male-to-male transmission → X-linked dominant pedigree**
- **Autism, large ears, and macroorchidism are physical exam findings present in Fragile X syndrome (an X-linked dominant condition)**

Section V - Hardy-Weinberg Principle

I. Overview

A. Used to estimate the allele and genotype frequencies in a population.

B. Can only be used to determine the frequency of one gene with multiple alleles (not multiple genes).

C. Assumptions include no natural selection, no mutation, no migration, random mating, and large populations.

II. Hardy-Weinberg Principle

A. Allele frequency: $p + q = 1$

1. p → frequency of the normal allele (A)
2. q → frequency of the mutant allele (a)

B. Genotype frequency: $p^2 + 2pq + q^2 = 1$

1. p^2 → frequency of individuals who are healthy (AA)
2. 2pq → carrier frequency (Aa)
3. q^2 → frequency of individuals with the disease (aa)

C. X-linked recessive diseases

1. $p + q = 1$
   a) p → frequency of healthy males (XY)
   b) q → frequency of males with the disease (XdY)
   c) The allele frequency for males and females will be identical (the p and q values for males will be the same in females)
2. $p^2 + 2pq + q^2 = 1$
   a) p^2 → frequency of females who are healthy (XX)
   b) 2pq → carrier frequency of females (XdX)
   c) q^2 → frequency of females with the disease (XdXd)

REVIEW QUESTIONS

1. A healthy 27-year-old female presents to the physician for genetic counseling with her husband. They would like to become pregnant in the near future, but have concerns that their offspring may develop cystic fibrosis. The wife's sister has cystic fibrosis, an autosomal recessive disorder with an incidence of approximately 1/90,000 in this particular population. The husband's history is noncontributory. What is the probability of the husband being a carrier?

    - **0.006587**
    - **The equation for genotype frequency ($p^2 + 2pq + q^2 = 1$) and with the equation for allele frequency ($p + q = 1$) must both be used to solve for the carrier frequency ($2pq$)**
    - **q2 (frequency of individuals with the disease) = 1/90,000**
    - **$q = \sqrt{1/90,000} = 1/300$**
    - **$p = 1 - q = 1 - 1/300 = 0.9967$**
    - **$2pq = 2(0.9967 \times 1/300) = 0.006587$**
    - **Alternatively, a shortcut can be used as follows:**
        - **The value of q is usually very small (i.e. 1/300) and because $p + q = 1$ we can conclude that p must approximate 1**
        - **Therefore, we can ignore the value of p (i.e. $2pq \sim 2q$)**
        - **$2q = 2(1/300) = 1/150 = 0.0066$ (notice that this is about the same as 0.006587)**

$p^2 + 2pq + q^2 = 1$ $\quad q^2 = 1/90,000$ $\quad p + q = 1$

$q = \sqrt{1/90,000}$ $\quad q = 1/300$ $\quad p = 1 - q$ $\quad p = 1 - 1/300$ $\quad p = 0.9967$

$2pq = 2(0.9967 \times 1/300)$

$2pq = 0.006587$

$p \sim 1 \quad 2pq \sim 2q \rightarrow 2(1/300) = 1/150 = 0.0066$

2. A healthy 27-year-old female presents to the physician for genetic counseling with her husband. They would like to become pregnant in the near future, but have concerns that their offspring may develop cystic fibrosis. The wife's sister has cystic fibrosis, an autosomal recessive disorder with an incidence of approximately 1/90,000 in this particular population. The husband's history is noncontributory. What is the probability of the couple having an affected child?

    - **1/900**
    - **From the prior question we know that the probability that husband is a carrier is 1/150**
    - **The wife's sister was affected so her parents must have been carriers**
    - **Because the wife is not affected (not aa) her probability of being a carrier is ⅔**
    - **The probability of a child getting both recessive alleles assuming both parents are carriers is ¼**
    - **1/150 x ⅔ x ¼ = 1/900**

Husband = 1/150

$1/150 \times 2/3 \times 1/4 = 1/900$

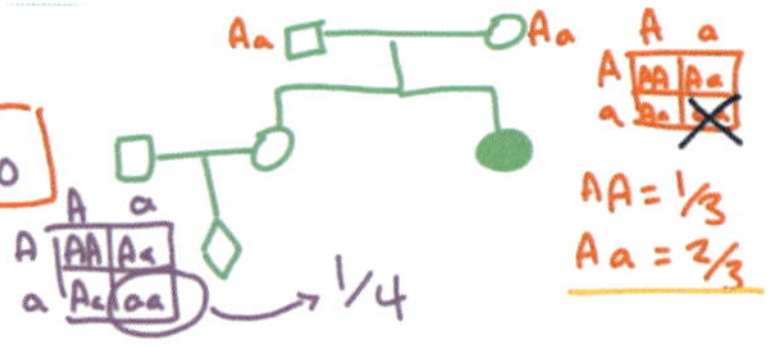

3. A 12-year-old boy has a history of easy bruising and severe joint swelling after minor injuries to his knees. This morning he underwent a dental procedure and has had continuous uncontrolled bleeding since that time. Hemophilia A is suspected. This is a disease that affects 1/10,000 males. Based on this information, what is the incidence of this disease among females in the same population?

    - **1/100,000,000**
    - **Hemophilia A is an X-linked recessive disease**
    - **In X-linked recessive diseases q represents the frequency of males with the disease**
    - **Males only have one X chromosomes so q = 1/10,000**
    - **Because the allele frequency is the same in males and females, we can conclude that q is also 1/10,000 for females**
    - **Females have two X chromosomes so they must have two diseased alleles in order to be affected by the disease**
    - **The frequency of affected females is q^2**
    - **$q^2 = 1/100,000,000$**

Section VI - Autosomal Dominant Diseases

I. Autosomal dominant diseases (Table 2.4.2)

A. Hypertrophic cardiomyopathy, Huntington disease, acute intermittent porphyria, von Hippel-Lindau disease, familial adenomatous polyposis, autosomal dominant polycystic kidney disease, hereditary spherocytosis, achondroplasia, Li-Fraumeni syndrome, von Willebrand disease, familial hypercholesterolemia, tuberous sclerosis, hereditary hemorrhagic telangiectasia, Marfan syndrome, neurofibromatosis type I, neurofibromatosis type II, multiple endocrine neoplasias osteogenesis imperfecta, and myotonic muscular dystrophy.

Disease	Cause	Findings	Notes
Achondroplasia	Fibroblast growth factor receptor 3 (FGFR3) mutation	-Chondrocyte proliferation impairment -Most common cause of dwarfism	-Autosomal dominant inheritance (15%) -Advanced paternal age (85%)
Acute intermittent porphyria	Porphobilinogen deaminase	-Abdominal pain, neuropathy, psychological disturbances -↑ urine porphobilinogen	-Results in defective heme synthesis → accumulation of toxic heme precursors
Neurofibromatosis type 1	NF1 gene mutation on chromosome 17	-Neurofibromas, café-au-lait spots, pheochromocytomas, optic gliomas, and pigmented iris hamartomas	-Exhibits variable expression but 100% penetrance
von Hippel-Lindau disease	Mutation of the VHL gene on chromosome 3	-Renal cell carcinoma, pheochromocytomas, hemangioblastomas	

Table 2.4.2 - Autosomal dominant diseases

REVIEW QUESTIONS

1. A 24-year-old male indicated by III,2 presents to the physician with his wife for genetic counseling prior to conception. He has a disorder characterized by impaired chondrocyte proliferation resulting in dwarfism. What was the most likely cause of hid disorder?

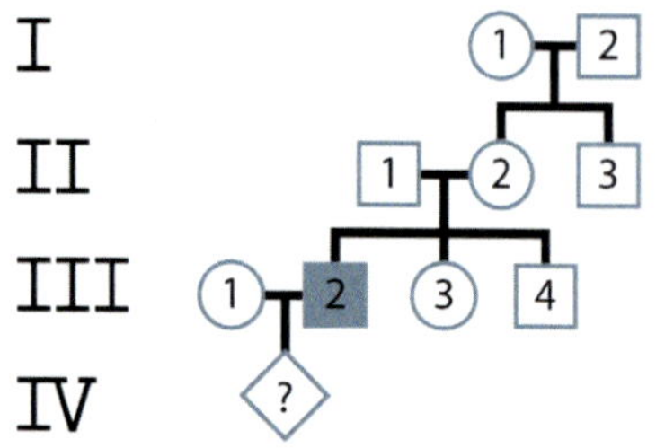

- **Advanced paternal age**
- **Impaired chondrocyte proliferation resulting in dwarfism → achondroplasia**
- **Most commonly caused by sporadic mutations in gametes due to advanced paternal age**
- **If the father indicated by II,1 was affected we could have concluded that the cause was due to autosomal dominant inheritance but this was not the case**

2. A 27-year-old female presents to the emergency department with a 3-hour history of abdominal pain and altered mental status. Several family members have presented in the past with similar problems. She states that she was at a party and consumed several alcoholic drinks when the pain began. Urine laboratory analysis reveals elevated porphobilinogen. What is most likely true of her condition?

   A) The pain typically starts at the periumbilical region and moves to McBurney's point
   B) A diagnosis can be made based upon an elevated serum lipase
   C) It results in defective heme synthesis
   D) The pain is typically worse after eating a fatty meal

- **Answer is C**
- **Multiple family members are affected hinting at the fact that the cause of her condition is genetic**
- **Urine analysis revealed elevated porphobilinogen → defective heme synthesis (acute intermittent porphyria)**
- **Acute intermittent porphyria is an autosomal dominant condition**

3. A 45-year-old male presents to the physician due to a 3-month history of heart palpitations, sporadic episodes of sweating, and intermittent headaches. Plasma metanephrines are elevated. Imaging of the abdomen reveals a renal mass. A biopsy is obtained followed by cytogenetic analysis which reveals a VHL gene mutation. What other malignancies are most likely associated with this patient's condition?

- **Renal cell carcinoma and hemangioblastomas**
- **This patient has a pheochromocytoma → heart palpitations, perspiration, headaches, HTN, and pallor (excess catecholamines cause a fight-or-flight response)**
- **The patient has a VHL gene mutation → he must have von Hippel-Lindau disease**
- **von Hippel-Lindau disease is associated with renal cell carcinoma and hemangioblastomas**

Section VI.1 - Autosomal Dominant Diseases

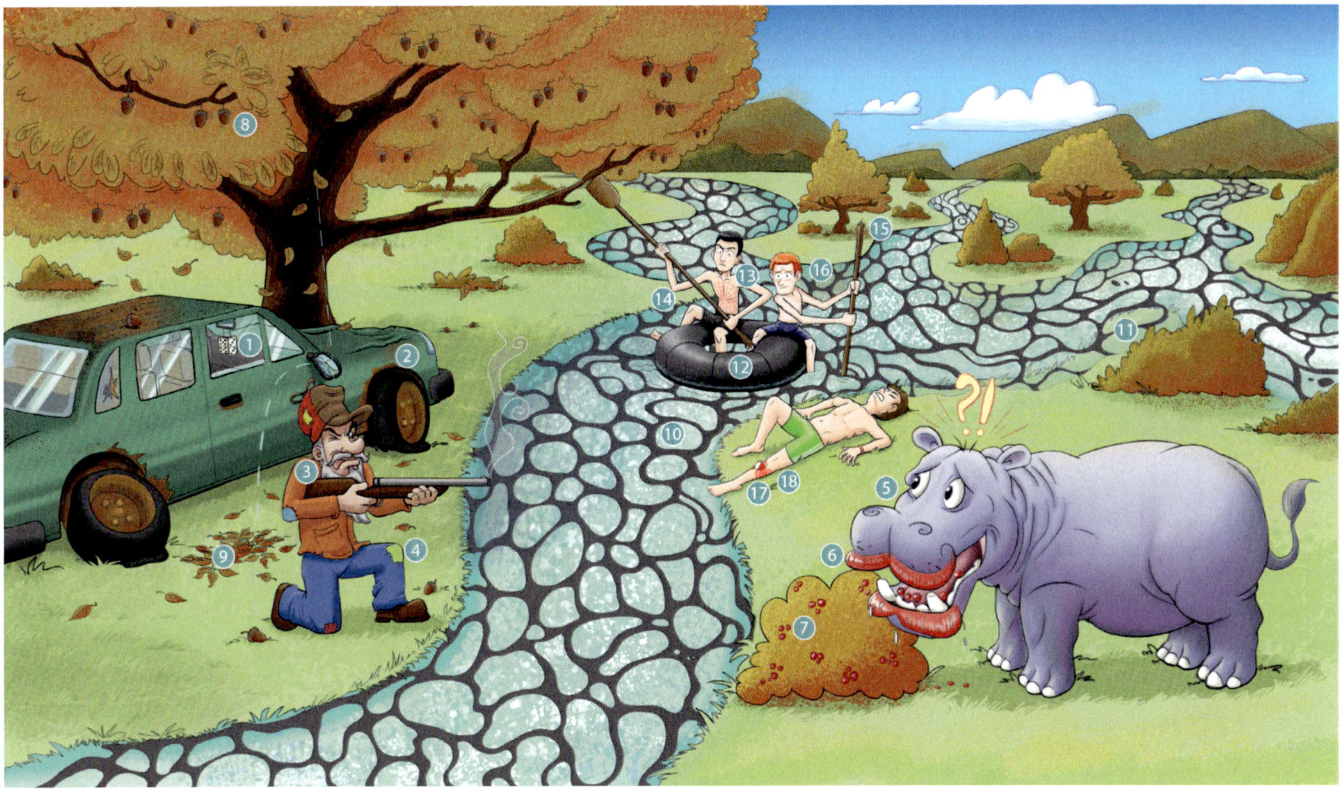

1. ______________________
2. ______________________
3. ______________________
4. ______________________
5. ______________________
6. ______________________
7. ______________________
8. ______________________
9. ______________________
10. ______________________
11. ______________________
12. ______________________
13. ______________________
14. ______________________
15. ______________________
16. ______________________
17. ______________________
18. ______________________

Section VII - X-linked Diseases

I. X-linked recessive diseases

Type	Diseases
X-linked recessive	Ornithine transcarbamylase deficiency, X-linked adrenoleukodystrophy, Duchenne and Becker muscular dystrophy, Hunter syndrome, ocular albinism, Bruton agammaglobulinemia, Wiskott-Aldrich syndrome, Lesch-Nyhan syndrome, Hyper-IgM syndrome, hemophilia A and B, severe combined immunodeficiency (SCID), Menkes disease, G6PD deficiency, and Fabry disease
X-linked dominant	Fragile X syndrome, hypophosphatemic rickets, and Alport syndrome
Other x-linked diseases	Rett syndrome

Table 2.4.3 - X-linked diseases

II. Muscular dystrophies (Figure 2.4.20)

A. Overview

1. Duchenne
2. Becker
3. Myotonic

B. Pathophysiology

1. Large gene → ↑ probability of spontaneous mutation
2. Dystrophin gene (DMD) mutation → frameshift or nonsense mutations → dystrophin protein dysfunction
3. Dystrophin is a protein present in muscle tissue that anchors actin to the extracellular matrix
4. Dystrophin dysfunction leads to myonecrosis

C. Clinical features

1. Progressive muscle weakness (lower and proximal limbs → upper and distal limbs)
2. Gower sign
3. Calf pseudohypertrophy (connective and adipose tissue replacement of muscle tissue)
4. Dilated cardiomyopathy
5. ↑ CK

D. Diagnosis

1. Molecular testing

E. Becker

1. Similar to Duchenne muscular dystrophy
2. Most commonly caused by none-frameshift mutations
3. Less severe because the dystrophin protein is more functional

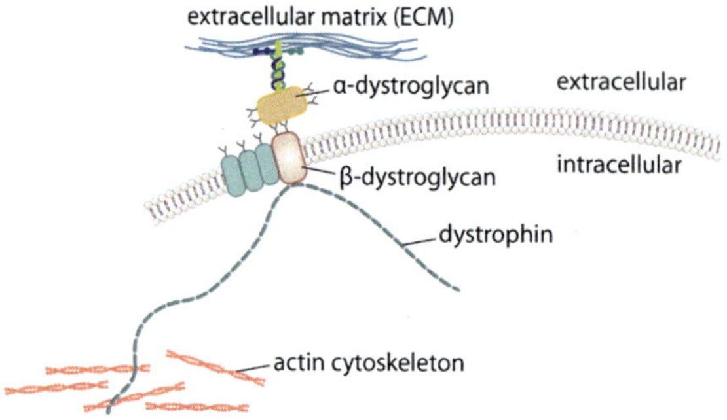

Figure 2.4.20 - Dystrophin

REVIEW QUESTIONS

1. A 4-year-old boy presents to the physician due to a 3-month history of muscle weakness. His mother states that when he lays on the ground he has to use his hands and arms to lift himself up. Physical exam reveals pseudohypertrophy of the calf muscles. Which of the following most likely represents the mode of inheritance of this patient's condition?

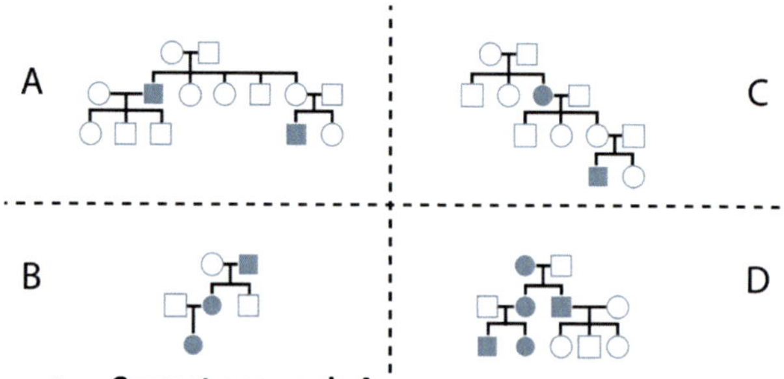

- **Correct answer is A**
- **"When he lays on the ground he has to use his hands and arms to lift himself up" is describing the Gower maneuver → muscular dystrophy**
- **Because he is less than 5 years old and his symptoms appear to be severe he most likely has Duchenne muscular dystrophy (an x-linked recessive condition)**
- **From the pedigrees only "A" represents an x-linked recessive disease (males are generally the only ones affected and there is no male-to-male transmission)**

Section VII.1 - X-linked Recessive Diseases

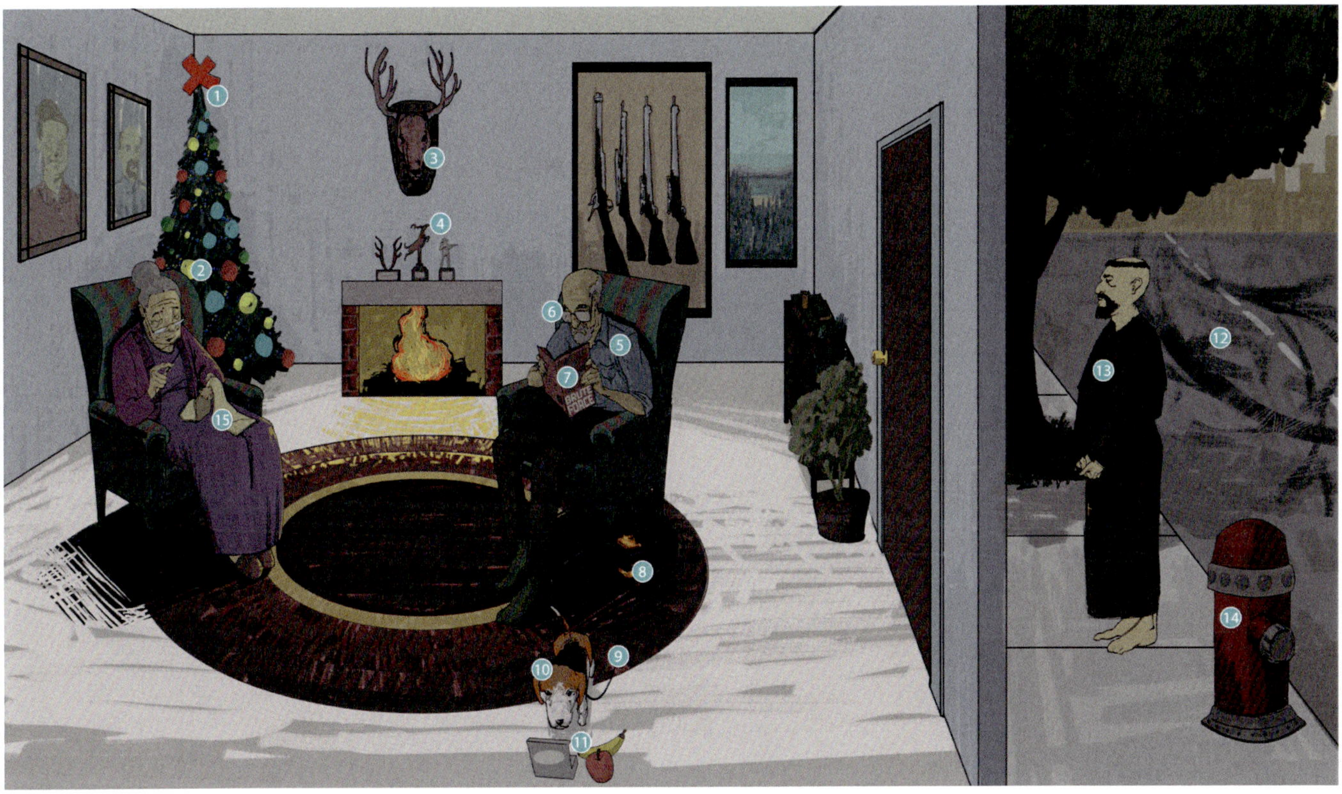

1. ______________________
2. ______________________
3. ______________________
4. ______________________
5. ______________________
6. ______________________
7. ______________________
8. ______________________
9. ______________________
10. ______________________
11. ______________________
12. ______________________
13. ______________________
14. ______________________
15. ______________________

Section VII.2 - Rett Syndrome

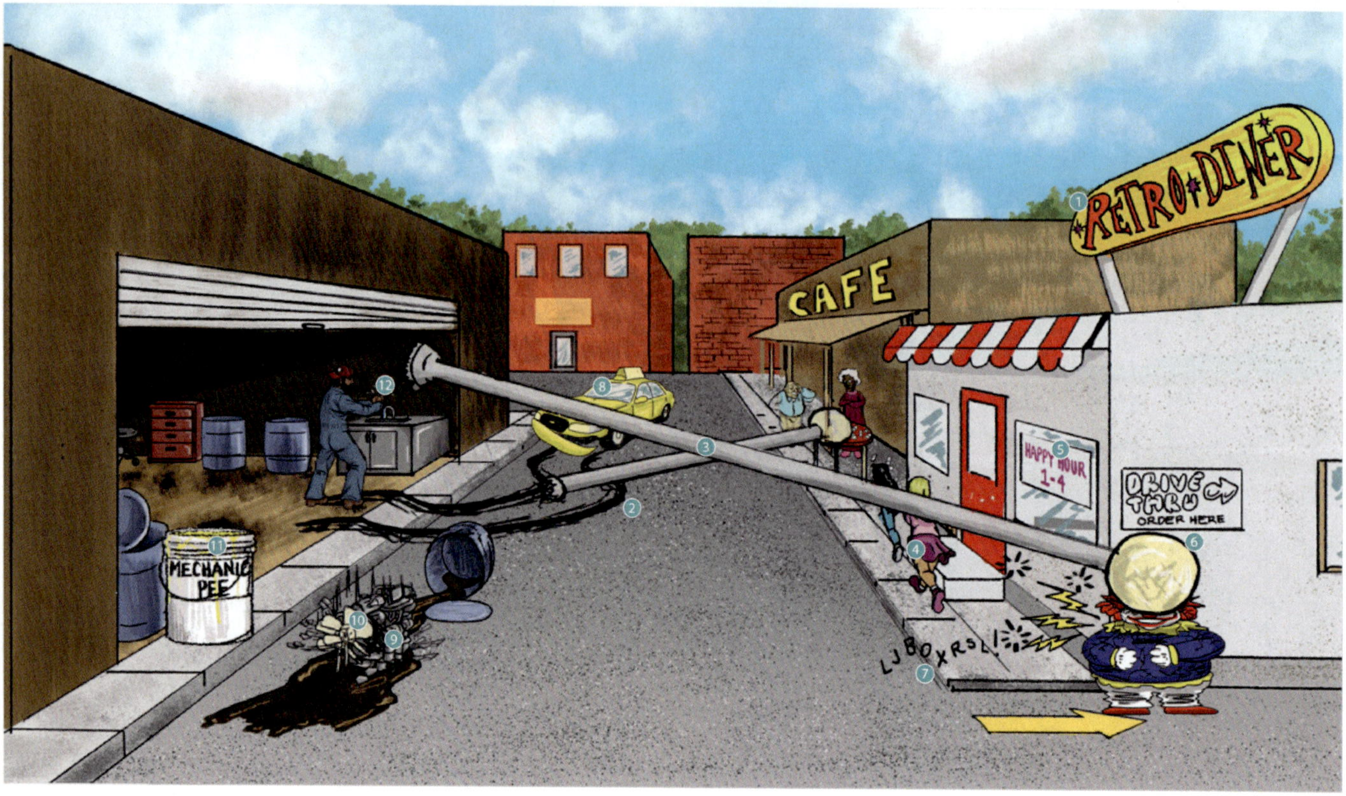

1. ______________________
2. ______________________
3. ______________________
4. ______________________
5. ______________________
6. ______________________
7. ______________________
8. ______________________
9. ______________________
10. ______________________
11. ______________________
12. ______________________

Section VIII - Autosomal Recessive Diseases

I. Autosomal recessive diseases

A. Albinism, Friedreich ataxia, glycogen storage diseases, hemochromatosis, mucopolysaccharidoses (not Hunter syndrome), sickle cell anemia, phenylketonuria, sphingolipidoses (not Fabry disease), Wilson disease, thalassemias, Kartagener syndrome, autosomal recessive polycystic kidney disease, cystic fibrosis

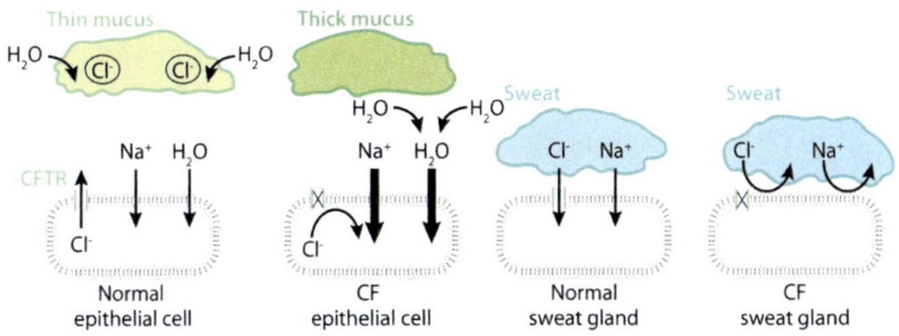

Figure 2.4.21 - Cystic fibrosis pathogenesis

II. Cystic fibrosis

A. Pathogenesis (Figure 2.4.21)

1. Autosomal recessive
2. Cystic fibrosis transmembrane regulator (CFTR) gene mutation
3. Deletion of Phe508
4. Secretes Cl^- in the GI tract and lungs
5. Reabsorbs Cl^- in the sweat glands
6. Mutation results in impaired glycosylation and folding of the CFTR protein → targeted for proteasomal degradation

B. Clinical features

1. Recurrent sinopulmonary infections (pseudomonas and staphylococcus aureus), bronchitis, and bronchiectasis
2. Male infertility (absent vas deferens → azoospermia)
3. Female infertility
4. Nasal polyps
5. Pancreatic insufficiency
6. Meconium ileus in newborns
7. Biliary and liver disease

C. Diagnosis

1. Elevated sweat chloride
2. Molecular testing
3. Nasal transepithelial potential difference
4. Immunoreactive trypsinogen

D. Treatment

1. Multifactorial (eg, chest therapy, antibiotics, pancreatic enzymes, lung transplant)
2. Lumacaftor and ivacaftor correct the misfolded CFTR protein and enhance the protein function once it reaches the plasma membrane

REVIEW QUESTIONS ?

1. How can infertility in men with cystic fibrosis be distinguished from infertility in men with Kartagener syndrome?
   - **In cystic fibrosis the vas deferens is blocked or absent resulting in azoospermia and infertility (no vas deferens).**
   - **In Kartagener syndrome, the sperm lack cilia so they unable to reach the oocyte (immotile).**

2. A 21-year-old Russian male presents to the physician with a fever, productive cough, and chest pain. He states that for most of his life he has lived in a rural area in Russia, but believes he has had multiple similar episodes that were undiagnosed. He also endorses fatty stools. On exam he has peripheral neuropathy. A chest x-ray is consistent with lobar pneumonia. Which of the following is most likely true of this patient's condition?

   A) Methylmalonic acid levels will be increased
   B) The condition will result in increased ubiquitin tagging of an abnormal protein
   C) The condition will improve if he eats more green vegetables
   D) The condition is associated with HLA-DQ2 and HLA-DQ8

   - **Correct answer is B**
   - **This patient has a history of recurrent pneumonia (multiple similar episodes that were undiagnosed), fatty stools, and peripheral neuropathy → cystic fibrosis**
   - **CF → pancreatic insufficiency → fat malabsorption → vitamin E deficiency → neuropathy**
   - **In cystic fibrosis the CFTR protein contains a mutation resulting in impaired glycosylation and proper folding of the protein**
   - **When proteins are not folded properly they're tagged by ubiquitin and then sent to the proteasome for degradation**

Section IX - Trinucleotide Repeat Disorders

I. Overview (Figure 2.4.22, Table 2.4.3)

A. Caused by an abnormal segment of repeated nucleotide bases within the genome

B. Anticipation is common

C. Mnemonic: "Try hunting for my eggs"

D. Huntington disease

E. Friedreich ataxia

F. Myotonic dystrophy

G. Fragile X syndrome

Disease	Inheritance	Repeat	Findings	Notes
Huntington disease	Autosomal dominant	$(CAG)_n$	- Repeats in the HTT gene on chromosome 4 - Basal ganglia atrophy → chorea, athetosis, aggression, depression, and dementia - Hydrocephalus ex vacuo - ↓ Ach, ↓ GABA, ↑ dopamine	CAG codes for glutamine → glutamine excitotoxicity "Caudate, Ach, and GABA"
Friedreich ataxia	Autosomal recessive	$(GAA)_n$	- Repeats in the FXN gene (codes for frataxin which is an iron binding protein) → mitochondrial dysfunction - Neurological deficits (lateral corticospinal tract, dorsal columns, spinocerebellar tract, and dorsal root ganglia) - Diabetes mellitus - Hypertrophic cardiomyopathy - Kyphoscoliosis in childhood - Feet deformities	"GAAit is ataxic"
Myotonic dystrophy	Autosomal dominant	$(CTG)_n$	- Repeats in the DMPK gene → myotonin protein kinase dysfunction - Muscle weakness, myotonia (prolonged muscle contraction), cataracts, gonadal atrophy, frontal balding, arrhythmias	"Cataracts, Tired muscles, Gonads"
Fragile X syndrome	X-linked dominant	$(CGG)_n$	- Repeats in the FMR1 gene → hypermethylation → silencing - Long face, large jaw, large ears, macroorchidism, neuropsychiatric changes (ADHD, autism, anxiety), mitral valve prolapse, joint hyperlaxity	Most common cause of inherited intellectual disability "Chin, Gonads, Gene silencing"

Table 2.4.4 - Trinucleotide repeat disorders

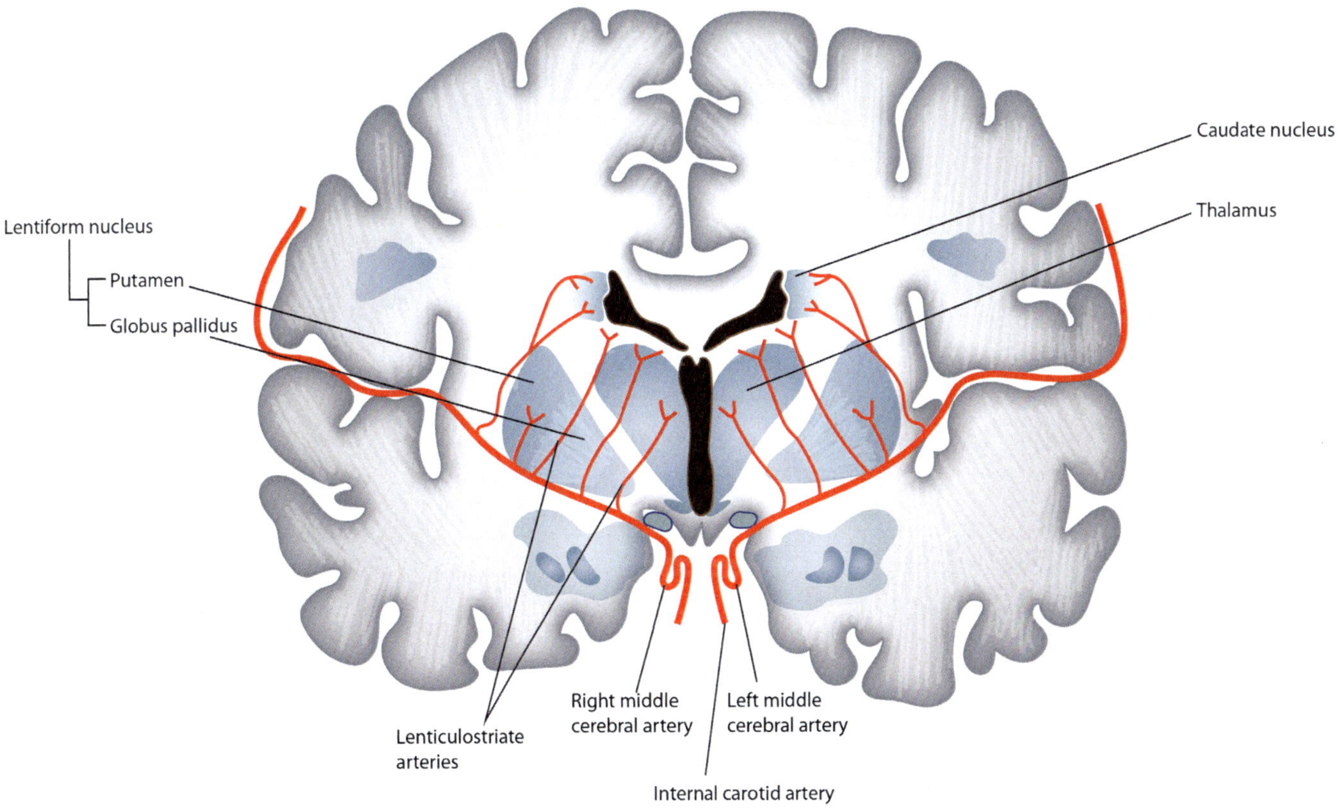

Figure 2.4.22 - Basal ganglia

REVIEW QUESTIONS

1. A 31-year-old male presents to the physician due to a 3-month history of depression and memory loss. An MRI of the brain reveals atrophy of the caudate. His father developed similar symptoms but at a much older age. What genetic principle explains these findings?

   - **Anticipation**
   - **This patient has depression, memory loss, and an MRI that shows atrophy of the caudate → Huntington disease**
   - **The development of symptoms at a much younger age compared to his father can be explained by anticipation (the tendency of a disease to occur earlier or to be more severe in succeeding generations)**

2. A 7-year-old boy with a history of anxiety presents to the physician for heart palpitations. On exam he has a murmur heard over the left sternal border. He also has a long face and large testes. PCR of the affected gene would most likely reveal what trinucleotide repeat?

   A) GAA
   B) CTG
   C) CAG
   D) CGG

   - **Correct answer is D**
   - **Anxiety, a cardiac murmur, a long face, and large testes → Fragile X syndrome**
   - **Fragile X syndrome is caused by CGG repeats**

Section IX.1 - Huntington Disease

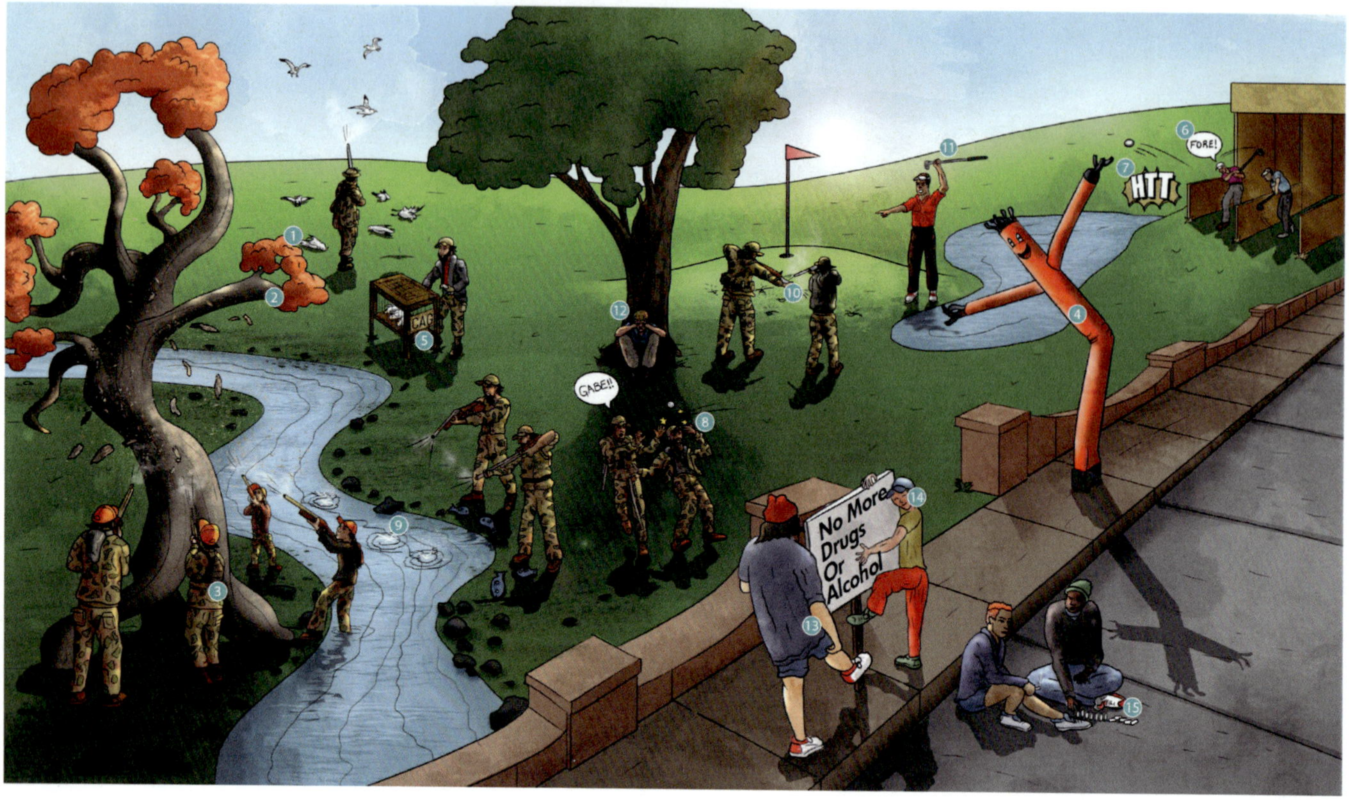

1. ______________________
2. ______________________
3. ______________________
4. ______________________
5. ______________________
6. ______________________
7. ______________________
8. ______________________
9. ______________________
10. ______________________
11. ______________________
12. ______________________
13. ______________________
14. ______________________
15. ______________________

Section IX.2 - Myotonic Dystrophy

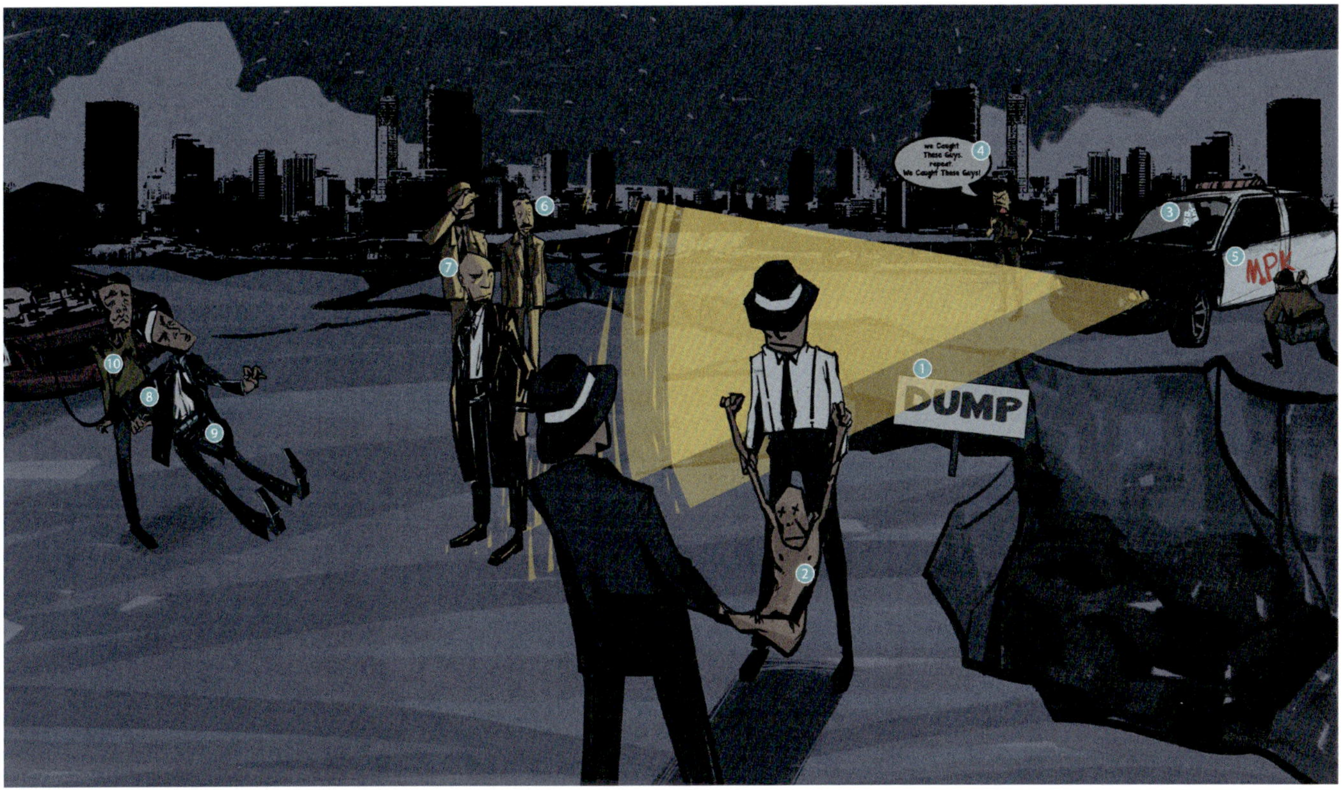

1. ______________________
2. ______________________
3. ______________________
4. ______________________
5. ______________________
6. ______________________
7. ______________________
8. ______________________
9. ______________________
10. ______________________

Section IX.3 - Fragile X Syndrome

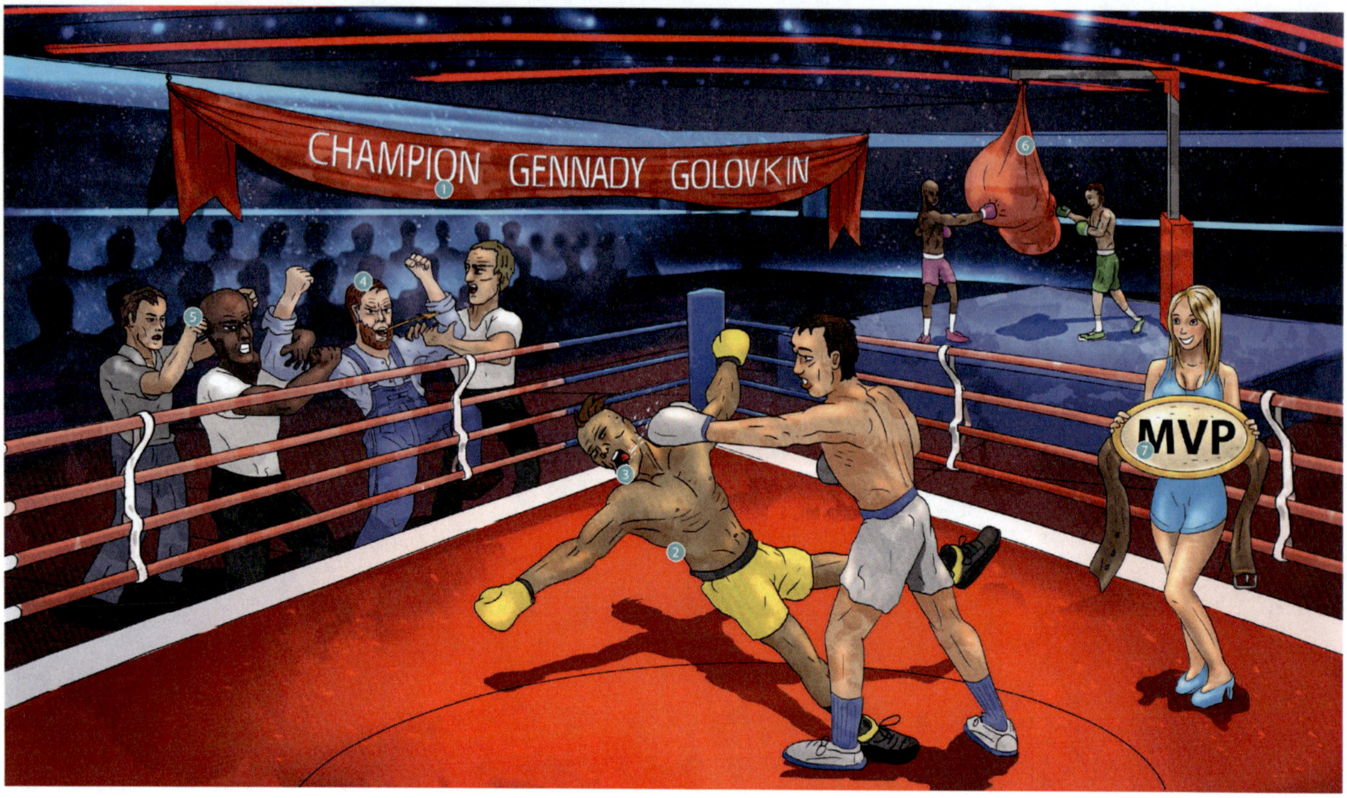

1. ______________________________
2. ______________________________
3. ______________________________
4. ______________________________
5. ______________________________
6. ______________________________
7. ______________________________

Section IX.4 - Friedreich Ataxia

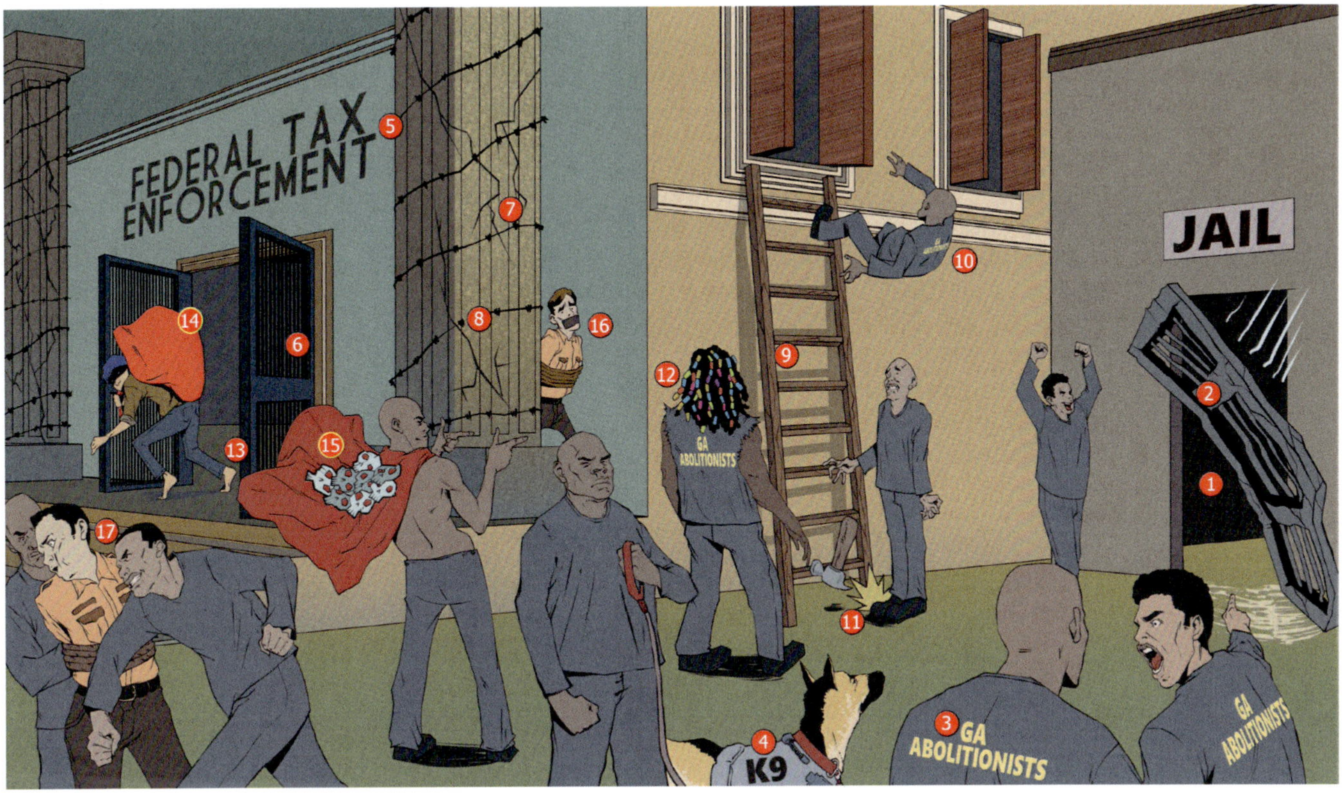

1. Freedom attack: Fredreich ataxia
2. Swaying gate: Staggering gait
3. GA Abolitionist: GAA repeat
4. K-9 unit: Chromosome 9
5. Federal tax: Frataxin gene
6. Iron bars: Iron binding protien
7. Cracked columns: Dorsal column degeneration
8. Spiny ceramic pillars: Spinocerebellar tract degeneration
9. Cracked ladder: Lateral
10. Falling off ladder: Frequent falling
11. Hammer falling on toe: Hammer toes
12. Dyed beads in hair: Diabetes mellitus
13. Tippy toes: Pes cavus
14. Heart-shaped bag: Hypertrophic cardiomyopathy
15. Cape with skulls: Kyphoscoliosis
16. Duct taped mouth: Dysarthria
17. Shaking eyes: Nystagmus

Section X - Autosomal Trisomies

Disease	Findings	Notes
Patau syndrome (trisomy 13)	-Intellectual disability -Congenital heart disease -Rocker bottom feet -Cleft lip and palate, microcephaly, microphthalmia, **polydactyly, polycystic kidney disease, cutis aplasia (small punched out round lesion on the scalp with an overlying thin membrane), omphalocele, holoprosencephaly**	-Death before 1
Edwards syndrome (trisomy 18)	-Intellectual disability -Congenital heart disease -Rocker bottom feet -Micrognathia (small jaw), prominent occiput, **low-set ears, clenched fists and overlapping fingers**	-Death before 1
Down syndrome (trisomy 21)	-Intellectual disability -Congenital heart disease -Flat facies, prominent epicanthal folds, upslanting palpebral fissures, small ears, **↑ skin at nape of neck, gap between 1st and 2nd toes, single palmar crease, Brushfield spots, Hirschsprung disease, duodenal atresia, ↑ risk of early-onset Alzheimer disease (chromosome 21 codes for amyloid precursor protein), ↑ risk of ALL and AML**	-First-trimester ultrasound may show a hypoplastic nasal bone and ↑ nuchal translucency -1% due to postfertilization mitotic error -4% due to unbalanced Robertsonian translocation (usually 14 and 21) -95% due to nondisjunction (↑ risk with advanced maternal age)

Table 2.4.5 - Autosomal trisomies

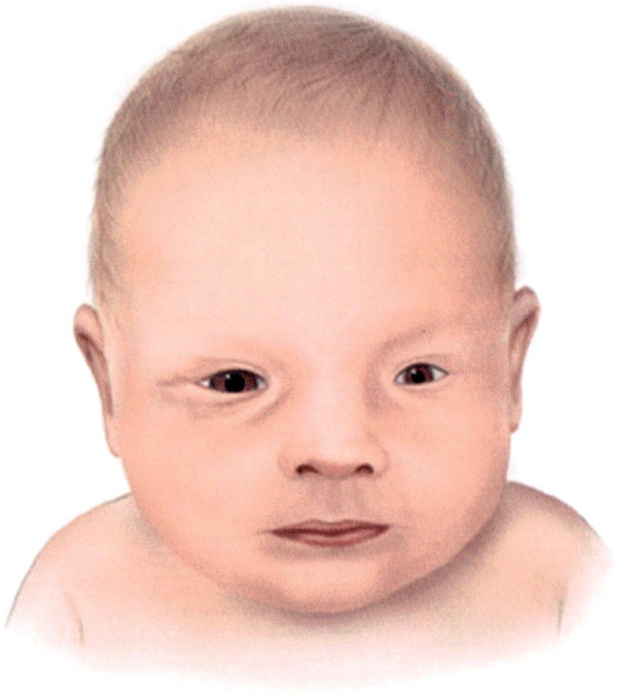

Photo Credit: Wikipedia/Public domain

Figure 2.4.23 - Microphthalmia

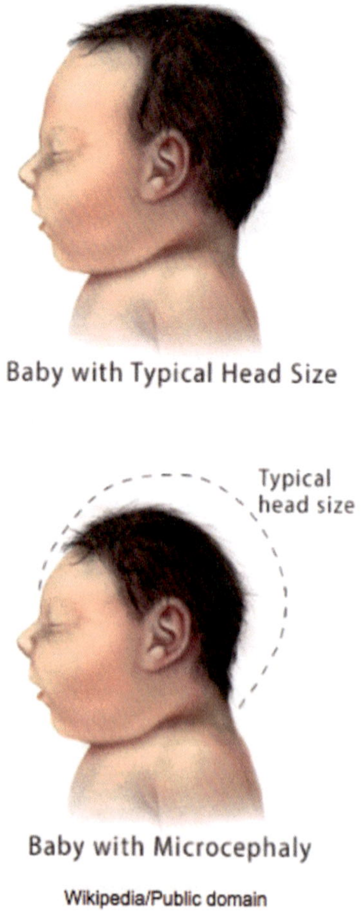

Photo Credit: Wikipedia/Public domain

Figure 2.4.24 - Microcephaly

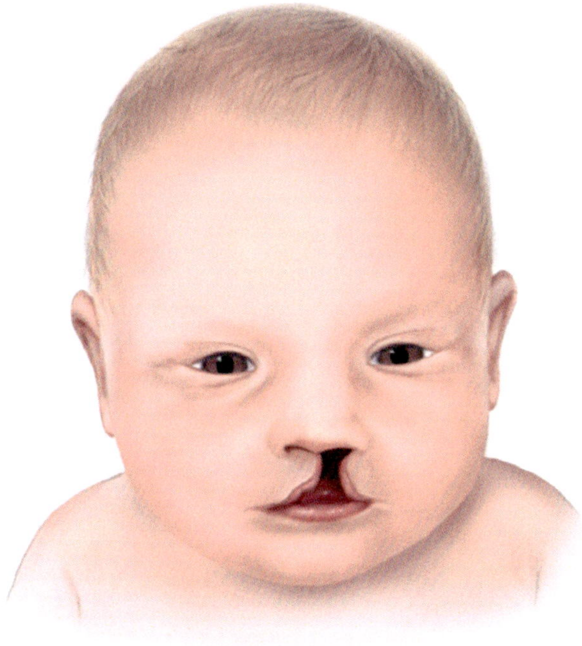

Photo Credit: Wikipedia/Public domain

Figure 2.4.25 - Cleft lip

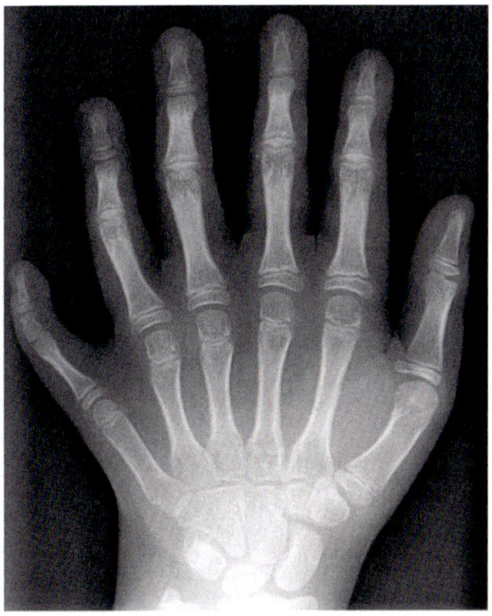

Photo Credit: By en:User:Drgnu23, subsequently altered by en:user:Grendelkhan, en:user: Raul654, and en:user:Solipsist. [GFDL (http://www.gnu.org/copyleft/fdl.html) or CC-BY-SA-3.0 (http://creativecommons.org/licenses/by-sa-3.0/)], from Wikimedia Commons

Figure 2.4.27 - Polydactyly

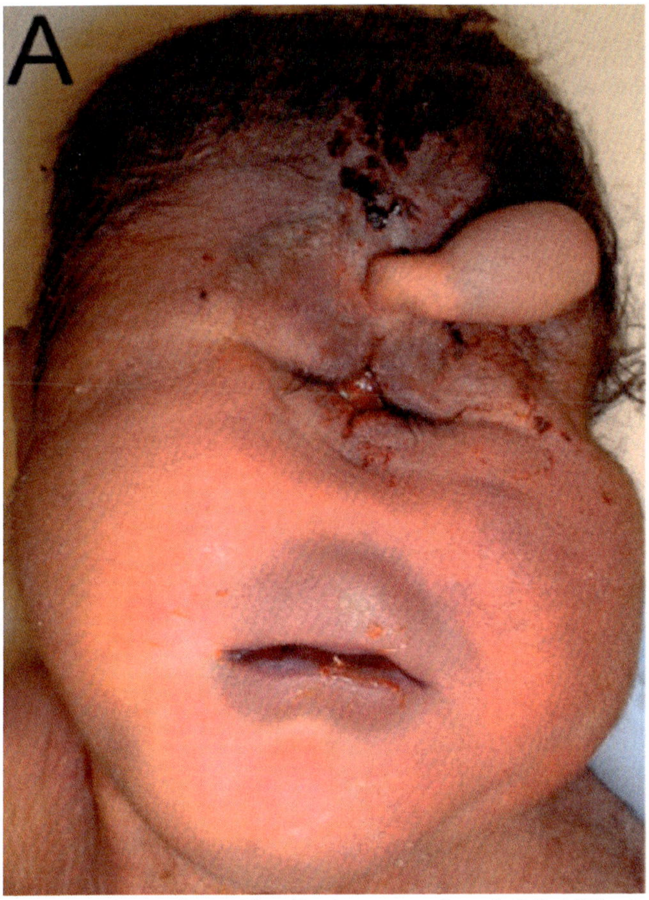

Photo Credit: By Chan A et al [CC BY 2.0 (https://creativecommons.org/licenses/by/2.0)], via Wikimedia Commons

Figure 2.4.26 - Holoprosencephaly

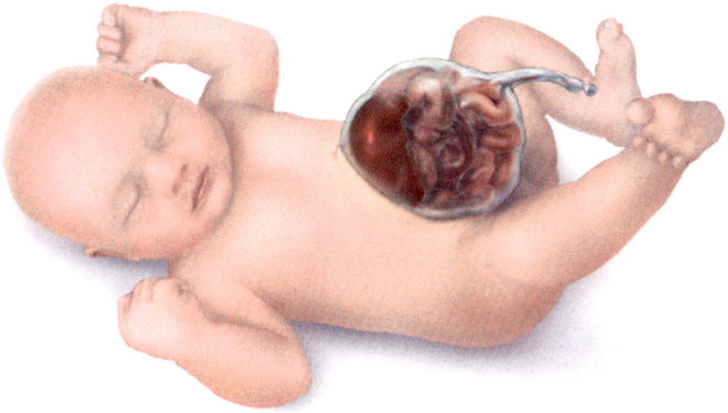

Photo Credit: Wikipedia/Public domain

Figure 2.4.28 - Omphalocele

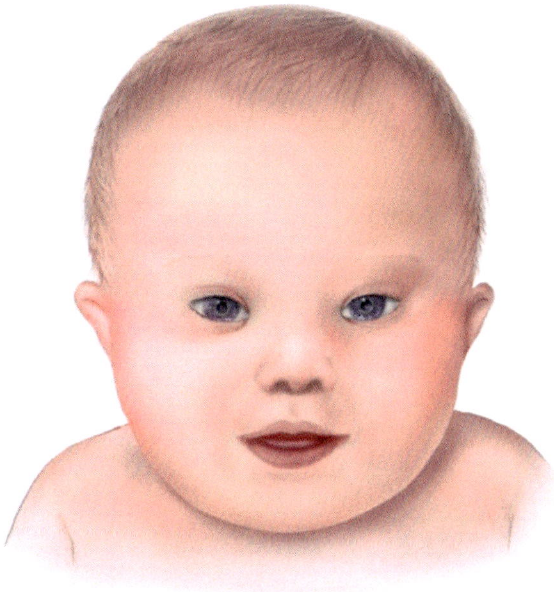

Wikipedia/Public domain

Photo Credit: Wikipedia/Public domain

Figure 2.4.29 - Down syndrome facial features

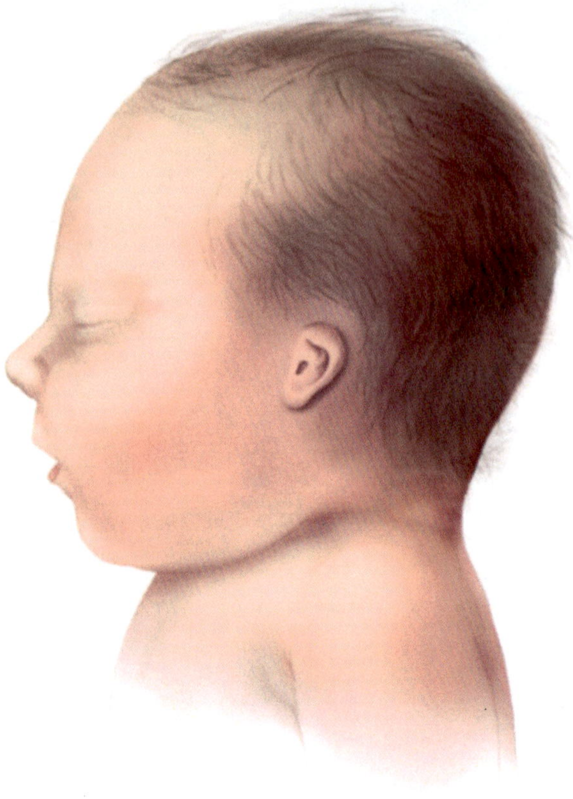

Photo Credit: Wikipedia/Public domain

Figure 2.4.30 - Small ears

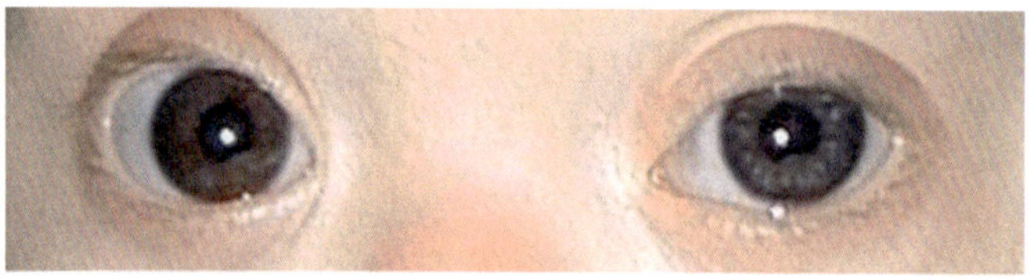

Photo Credit: By Szmon Tomczak was the original author of this photo, [CC0], via Wikimedia Commons

Figure 2.4.31 - Brushfield spots

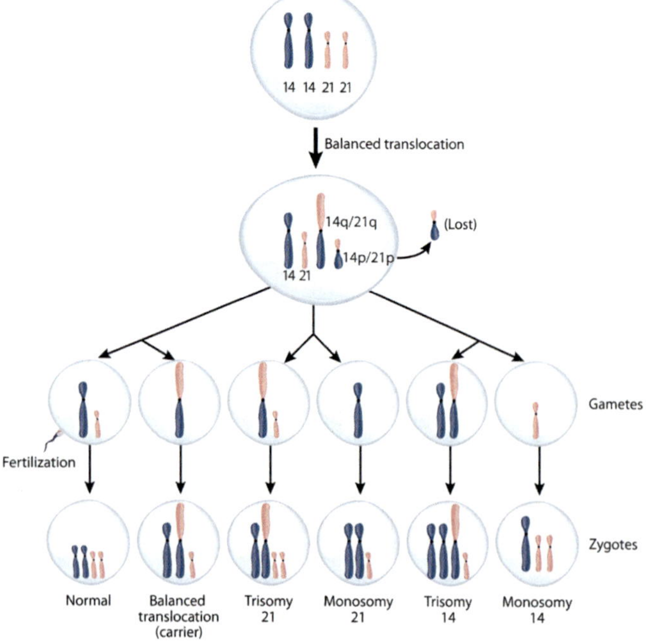

Figure 2.4.32 - Robertsonian translocation

REVIEW QUESTIONS ?

1. A healthy 26-year-old female delivers a male at term. In the delivery room he is examined and found to have flat facies, a gap between the 1st and 2nd toes, and a cardiac murmur. What karyotype is most consistent with this patient's condition?

   A) 47, XXY
   B) 47, XY, +13
   C) 47, XY, +18
   D) 46, XY, t(11;14)
   E) 46, XY, t(14;21)

- **Correct answer is E**
- **Flat facies, a gap between the 1st and 2nd toes, and a cardiac murmur → Down syndrome**
- **A Robertsonian translocation between chromosomes 14 and 21 could cause Down syndrome → 46, XY, t(14;21)**

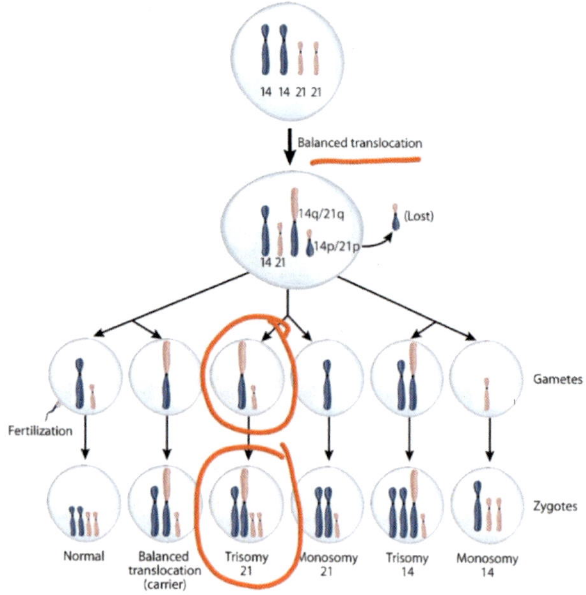

Section X.1 - Down Syndrome

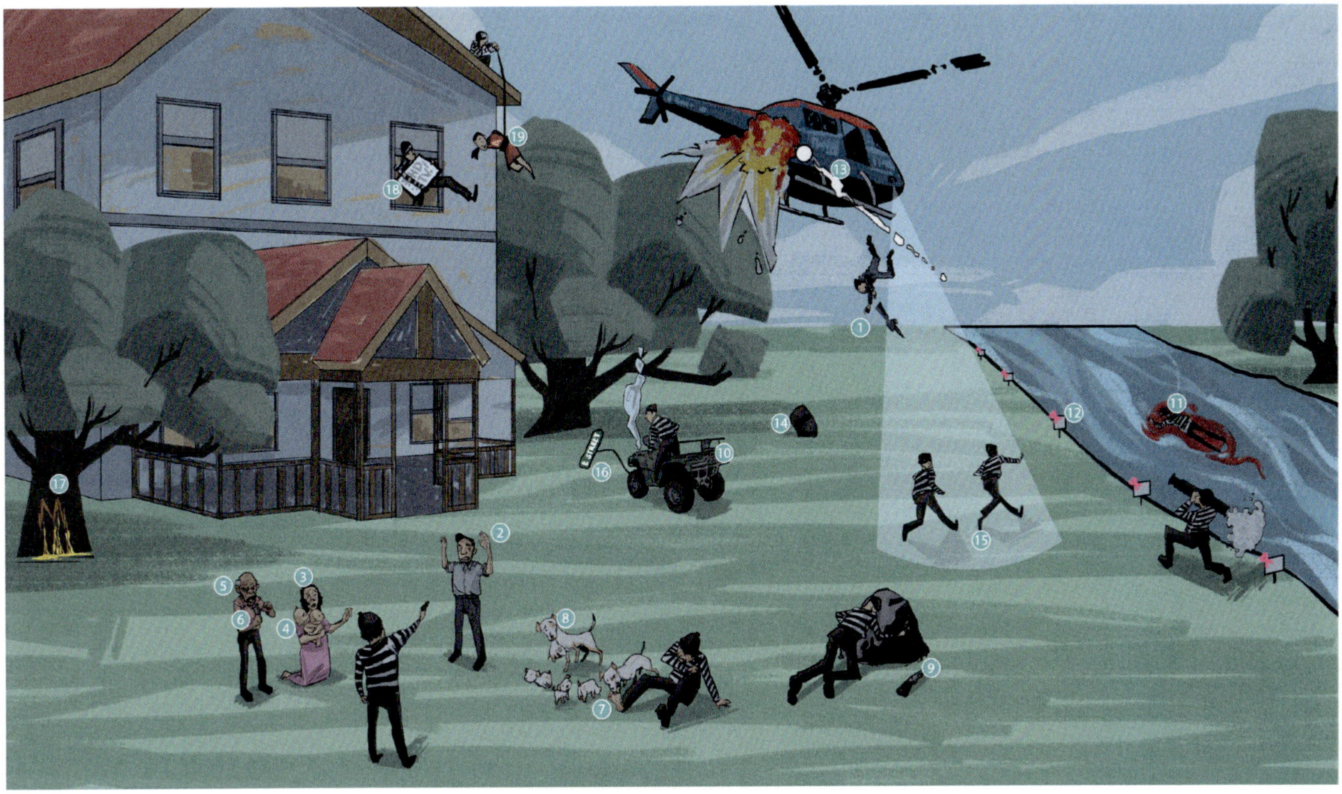

1. ______________________
2. ______________________
3. ______________________
4. ______________________
5. ______________________
6. ______________________
7. ______________________
8. ______________________
9. ______________________
10. ______________________
11. ______________________
12. ______________________
13. ______________________
14. ______________________
15. ______________________
16. ______________________
17. ______________________
18. ______________________
19. ______________________

Section X.2 - Edwards Syndrome

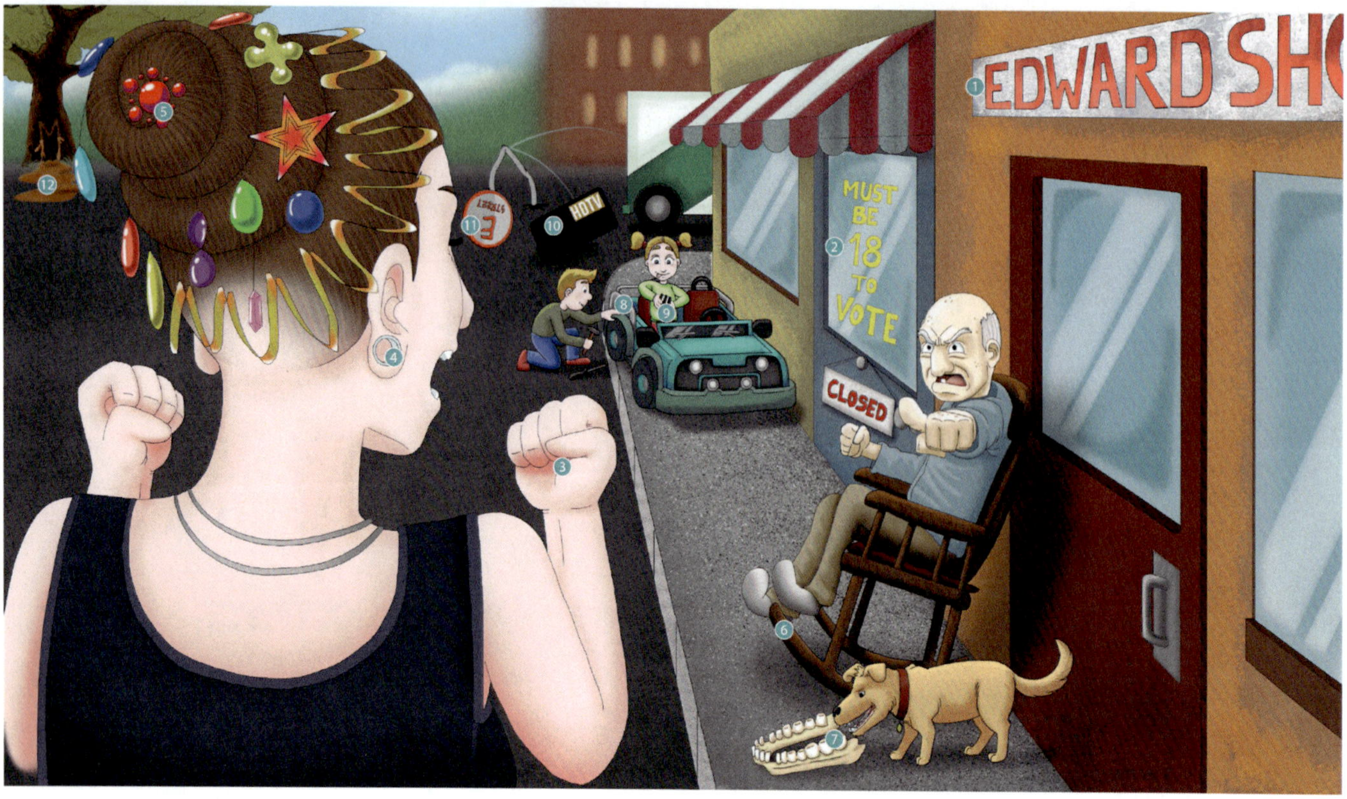

1. ______________________
2. ______________________
3. ______________________
4. ______________________
5. ______________________
6. ______________________
7. ______________________
8. ______________________
9. ______________________
10. ______________________
11. ______________________
12. ______________________

Section X.3 - Patau Syndrome

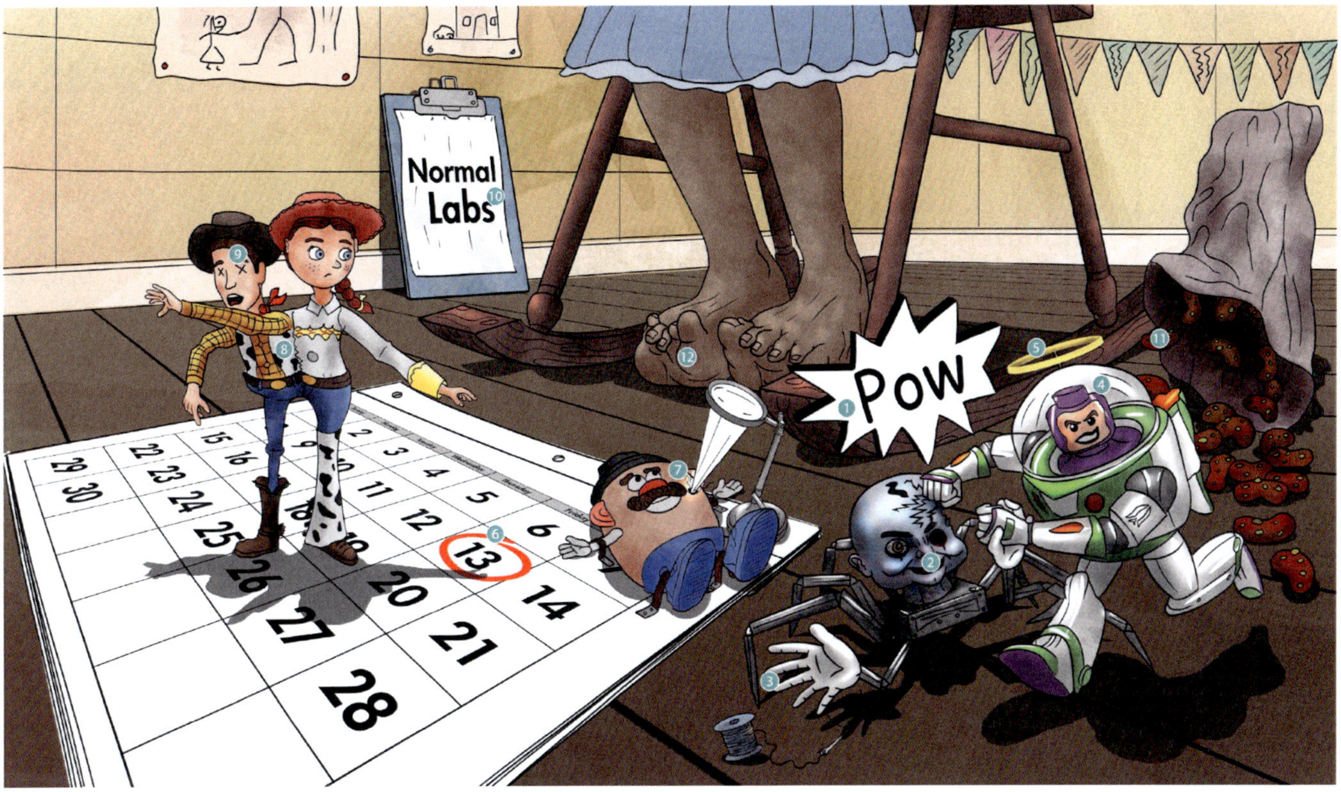

1. ______________________
2. ______________________
3. ______________________
4. ______________________
5. ______________________
6. ______________________
7. ______________________
8. ______________________
9. ______________________
10. ______________________
11. ______________________
12. ______________________

Section XI - Sex Chromosome Disorders

Disease	Karyotype	Cause	Findings	Labs
Klinefelter syndrome	47, XXY	-Nondisjunction -Mosaicism (rare)	- Testicular fibrosis/atrophy, infertility, eunuchoid body shape, gynecomastia, **mild intellectual disability (uncommon), tall, long extremities** -Barr body present due to inactivated X chromosome	- Testicular fibrosis → ↓ inhibin B (Sertoli cells), ↓ testosterone (Leydig cells) → ↑ FSH, ↑ LH
Turner syndrome	45, XO	-Nondisjunction -Mosaicism	- Ovarian dysgenesis (streak ovaries), menopause before menarche, shield chest (widely spaced nipples and underdeveloped breasts), **short stature, preductal coarctation, bicuspid aortic valve, cystic hygroma, webbed neck, lymphedema, horseshoe kidney** - Pregnancy possible with in vitro fertilization (ovum must be provided by someone else) -Absent Barr body	- Ovarian dysgenesis → ↓ estrogen → ↑ FSH and LH
XYY syndrome (double Y males)	47, XYY	-Nondisjunction	- Usually not diagnosed due to normal phenotype - Tall, mild learning disability, autism, severe acne	- Normal

Table 2.4.6 - Sex chromosome disorders

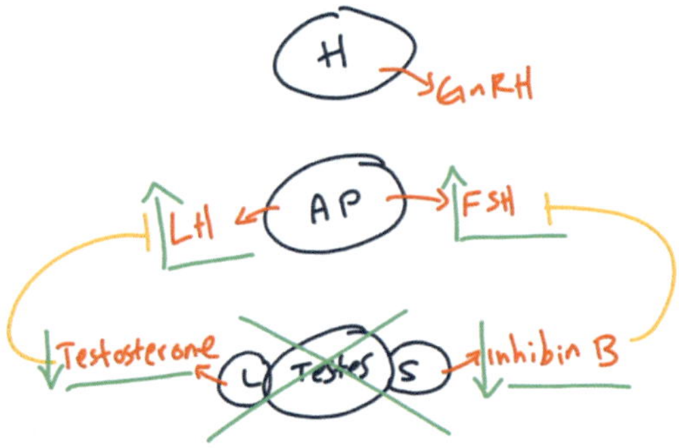

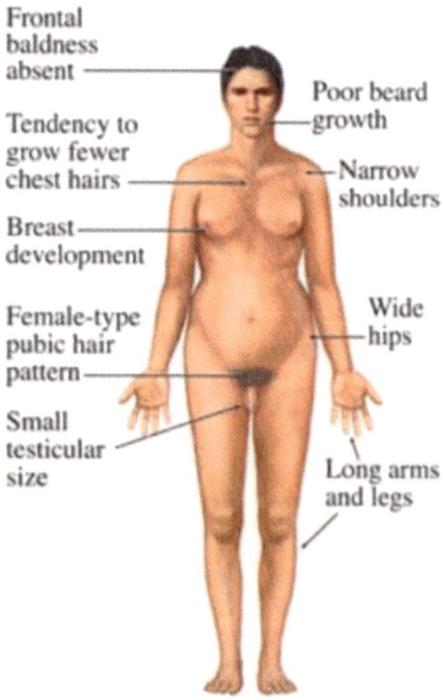

Photo Credit: http://smithperiod6.wikispaces.com/Klinefelter's+Syndrome [CC BY-SA 3.0 (https://creativecommons.org/licenses/by-sa/3.0) or Attribution], via Wikimedia Commons

Figure 2.4.33 - Klinefelter syndrome

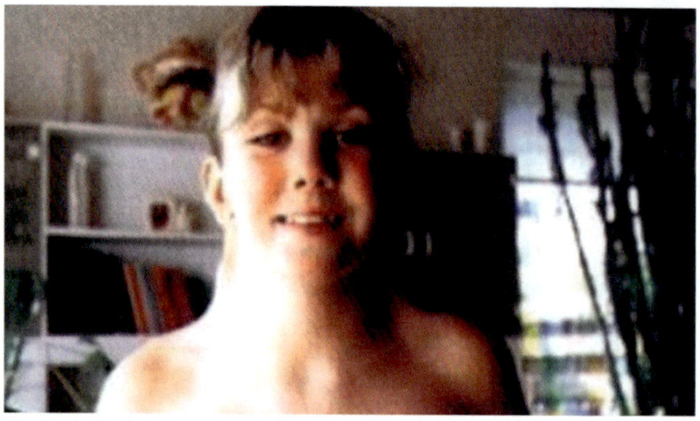

Photo Credit: By Johannes Nielsen (http://www.aaa.dk/TURNER/ENGELSK/TURN_ORI.HTM#baby) [CC BY 2.0 (https://creativecommons.org/licenses/by/2.0)], via Wikimedia Commons

Figure 2.4.34 - Webbed neck

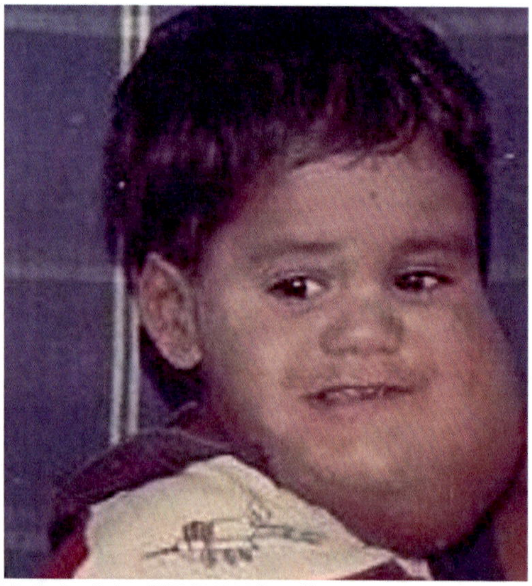

Photo Credit: By Vardhan Kothapalli [CC BY-SA 3.0 (https://creativecommons.org/licenses/by-sa/3.0)], from Wikimedia Commons

Figure 2.4.35 - Cystic hygroma

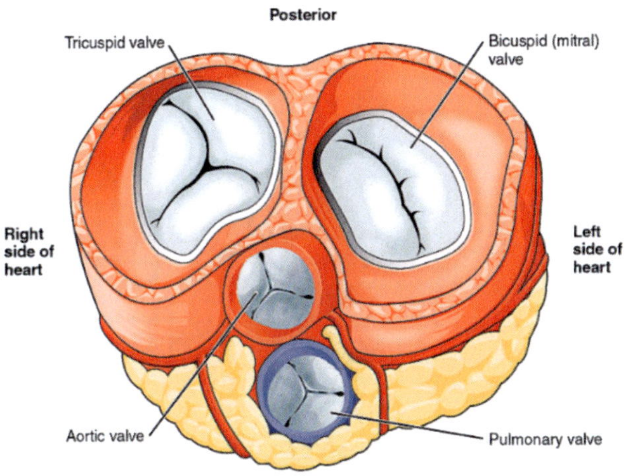

Photo Credit: By OpenStax College [CC BY 3.0 (https://creativecommons.org/licenses/by/3.0)], via Wikimedia Commons

Figure 2.4.36 - Bicuspid and tricuspid valves

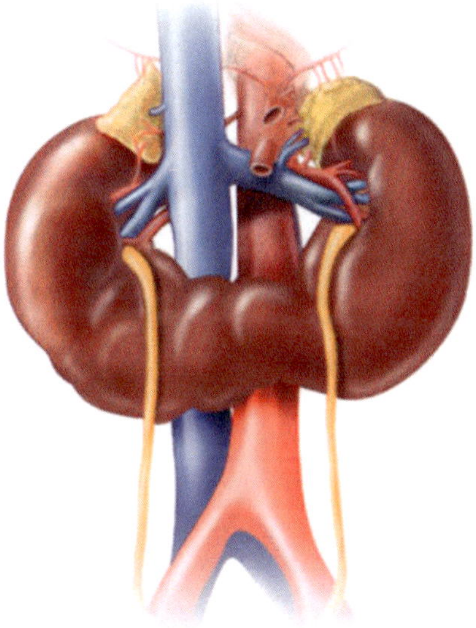

Photo Credit: By Prosyannikov (http://03uro.ru/uropedia/horseshoe-kidney) [CC BY-SA 2.5 (https://creativecommons.org/licenses/by-sa/2.5)], via Wikimedia Commons

Figure 2.4.37 - Horseshoe kidney

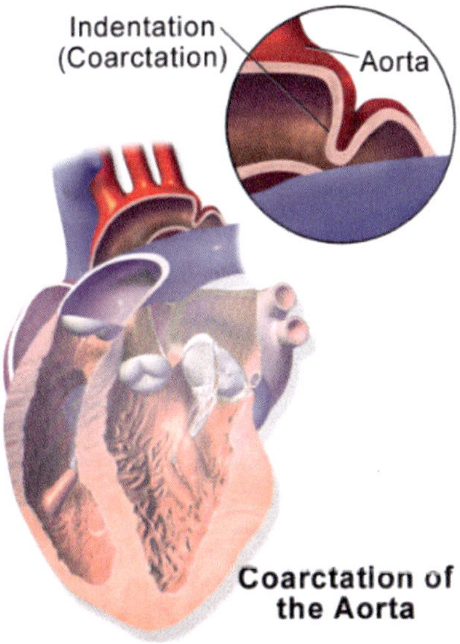

Photo Credit: By CruceBlaus. Blausen.com staff (2014). "Medical gallery of Blausen Medical 2014". WikiJournal of Medicine 1 (2). DOI10. 15347/wjm/2014.010. ISSN 2002-4436. [CC BY 3.0 (https://creativecommons.org/licenses/by-sa/3.0)], from Wikimedia Commons

Figure 2.4.38 - Coarctation of the aorta

REVIEW QUESTIONS

1. A 27-year-old male presents to the physician with his wife due to infertility problems. They state that they have been attempting to become pregnant for two years without success. Physical exam reveals a tall man with small testes. Laboratory findings include elevated levels of FSH and LH. What is the most likely diagnosis?
   - **Klinefelter syndrome**
   - **Infertility in a tall man with small testes → Klinefelter syndrome**
   - **↑ FSH and LH are due to fibrosis of the testes**

2. A 17-year-old girl presents to the physician with concerns regarding menstruation. She endorses amenorrhea and is concerned that there may be something wrong. On exam she has widely spaced nipples and underdeveloped breasts. Which of the following is most likely present in this individual?

   A) Diminished femoral pulses
   B) Bicuspid pulmonic valve
   C) Intellectual disability
   D) Decreased follicle stimulating hormone levels

   - **Correct answer is A**
   - **Amenorrhea, widely spaced nipples, and underdeveloped breasts → Turner syndrome**
   - **Turner syndrome is associated with coarctation of the aorta → diminished femoral pulses (A)**
   - **This occurs because the blood flow traveling to the lower extremities is impaired**

Section XI.1 - Turner Syndrome

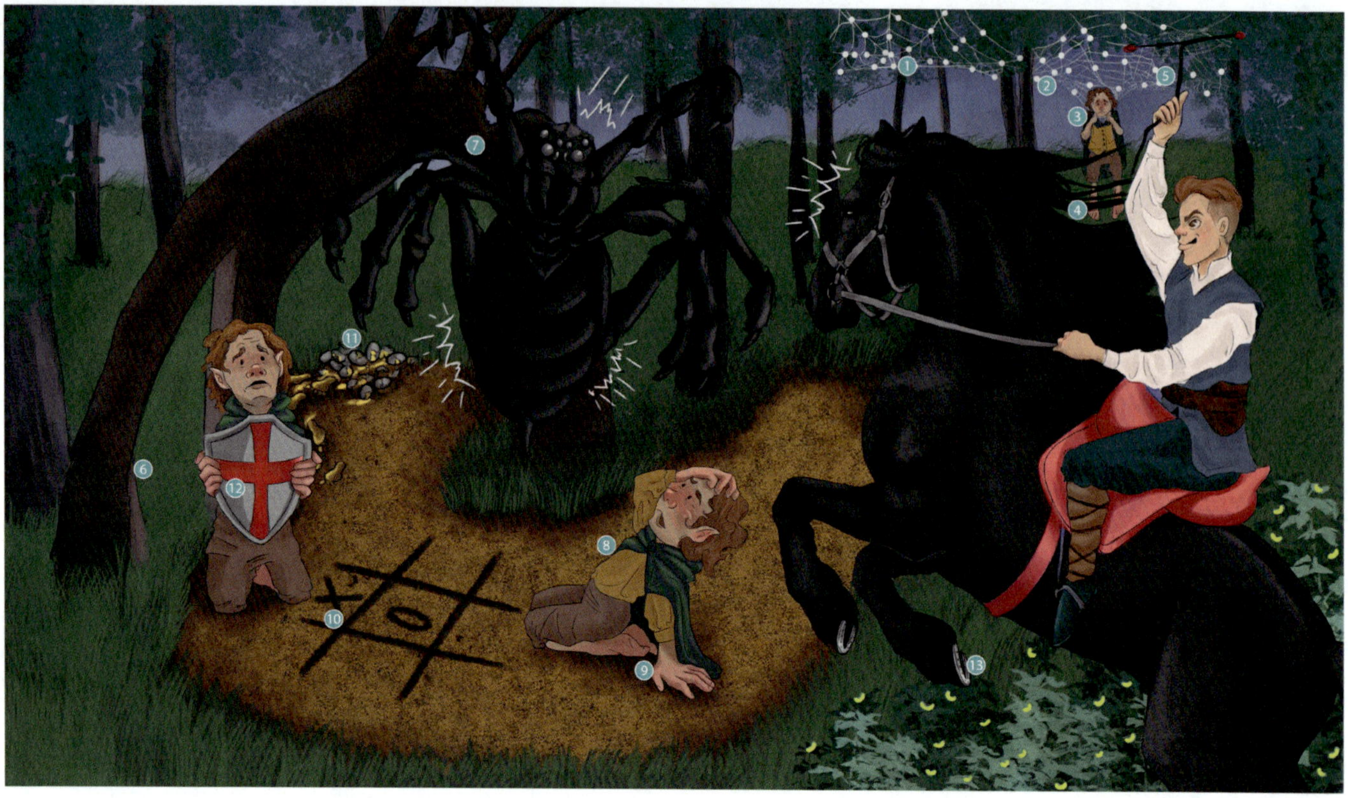

1. ______________________
2. ______________________
3. ______________________
4. ______________________
5. ______________________
6. ______________________
7. ______________________
8. ______________________
9. ______________________
10. ______________________
11. ______________________
12. ______________________
13. ______________________

Section XI.2 - Klinefelter Syndrome

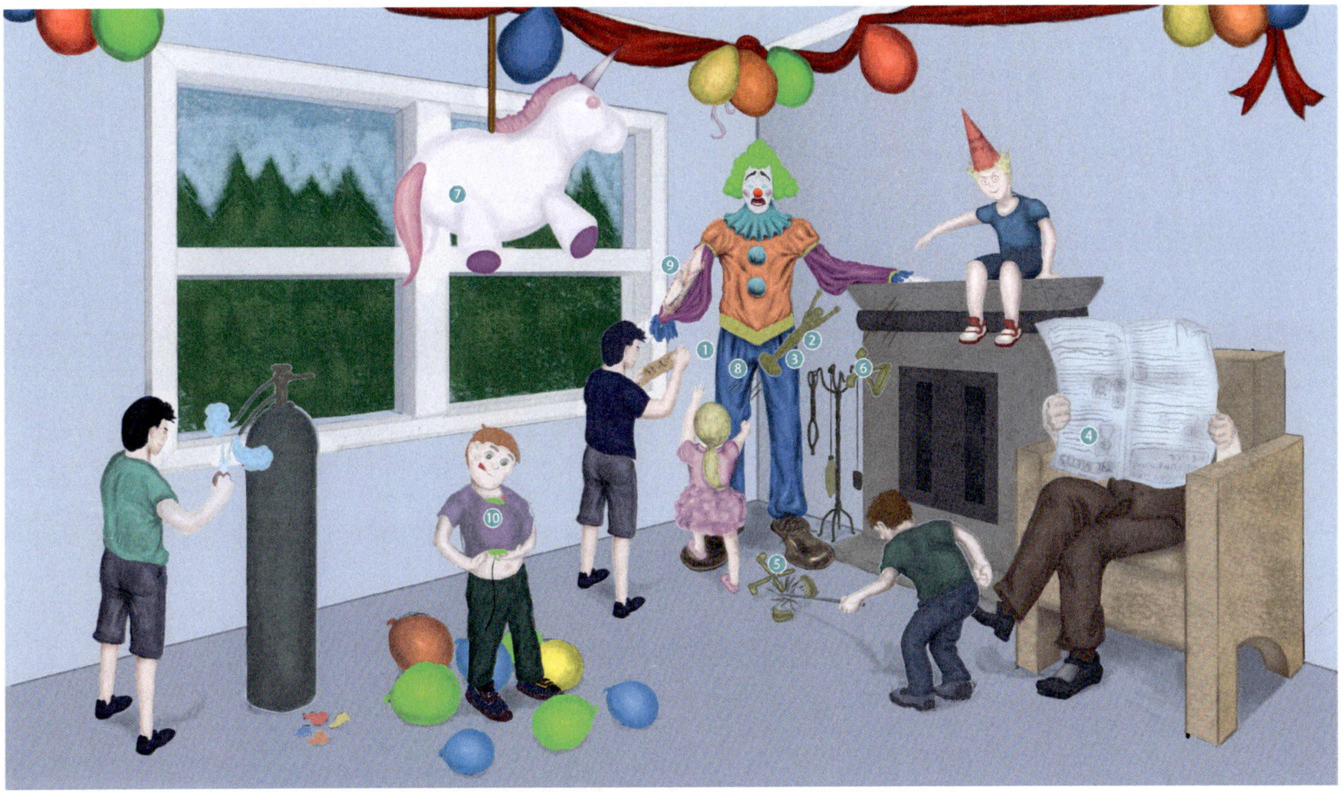

1. ______________________
2. ______________________
3. ______________________
4. ______________________
5. ______________________
6. ______________________
7. ______________________
8. ______________________
9. ______________________
10. ______________________

Section XII - Deletion syndromes

I. Overview (Table 2.4.7)

A. An entire segment of a chromosome is deleted

B. Due to homologous recombination errors during meiosis

C. Cri-du-chat syndrome

D. Williams syndrome

Disease	Pathophysiology	Findings	Notes
Cri-du-chat syndrome	Deletion of a segment of the short arm of chromosome 5	-High-pitched cry (similar to a cat), intellectual disability, microcephaly, congenital heart disease (VSD), epicanthal folds	Cri du chat: cry of the cat
Williams syndrome	Deletion of a segment of the long arm of chromosome 7 (includes elastin gene)	-"Elfin" appearance, intellectual disability, extremely friendly, well-developed verbal skills, congenital heart disease (supravalvular aortic stenosis), renal artery stenosis, hypercalcemia (↑ vitamin D sensitivity)	"Will Ferrell in the Elf is very friendly"
DiGeorge syndrome (velocardiofacial syndrome)	Deletion of a segment of the long arm of chromosome 22 (22q11) → aberrant development of the 3rd and 4th pharyngeal pouches (thymus, parathyroid glands, pharynx, upper portion of the heart)	-Cleft palate, abnormal facial features (hypertelorism), thymic aplasia (↓ T-cells → immunodeficiency), cardiac defects (tetralogy of Fallot, truncus arteriosus, ASD, VSD, aortic arch defects), hypocalcemia -Absent thymic shadow on x-ray	"CATCH-22"

Table 2.4.7 - Microdeletion syndromes

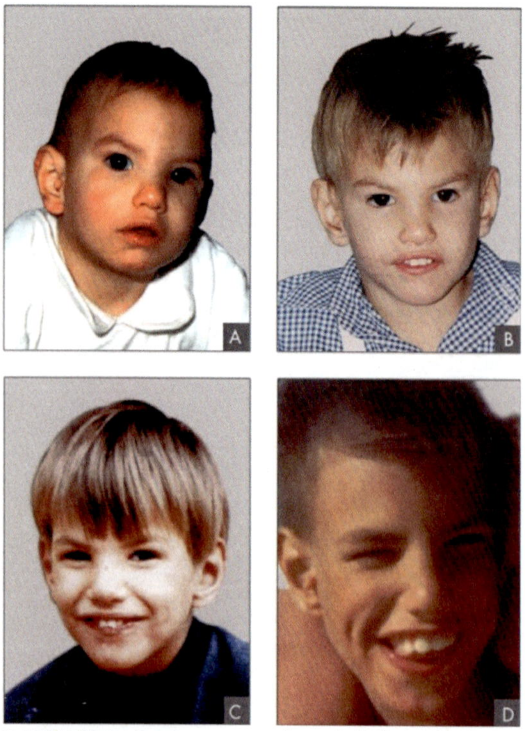

Figure 2.4.39 - Cri-du-chat syndrome

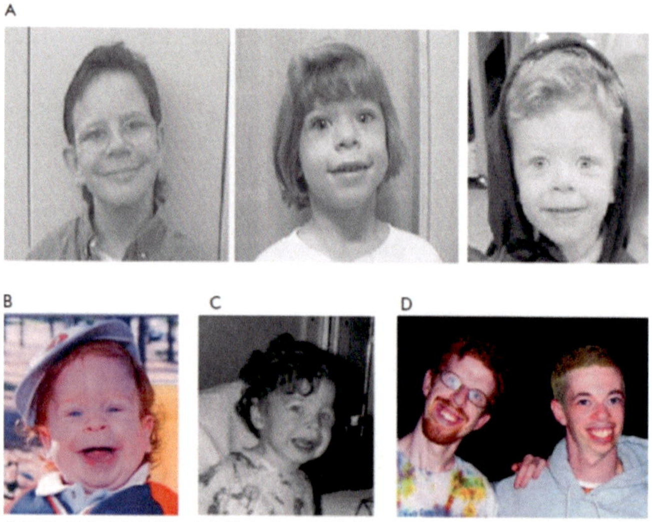

Figure 2.4.40 - Williams syndrome

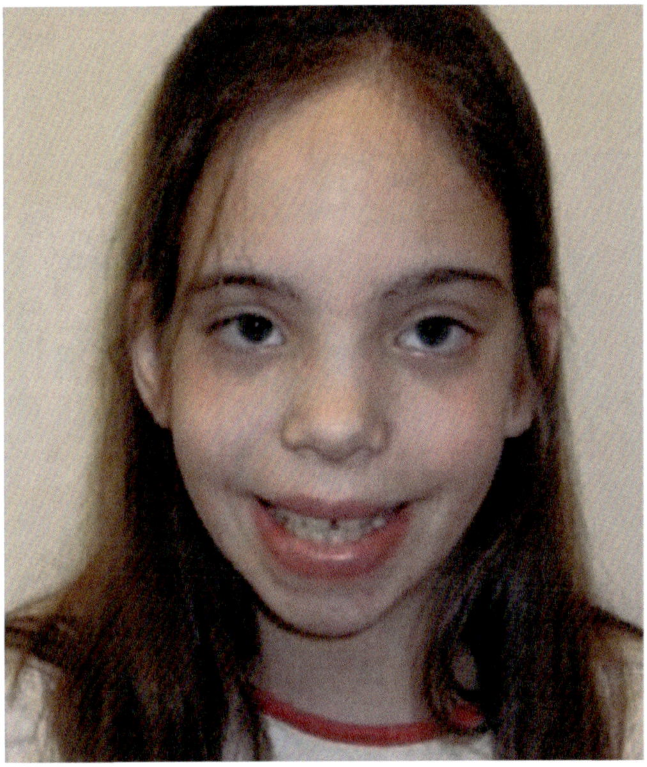

Photo Credit: By Nicole R Tartaglia, corresponding author 1,2 Susan Howell, 1,2 Ashley Sutherland, 1 Rebecca Wilson, 2 and Lennie Wilson 3 [CC BY 2.5 (https://creativecommons.org/licenses/by/2.5)], via Wikimedia Commons

Figure 2.4.41 - Hypertelorism

REVIEW QUESTIONS

1. A healthy 24-year-old female delivers a male at term. In the delivery room he is examined and found to have a cleft lip, cleft palate, a cardiac murmur, and hypertelorism. Which of the following is most likely true of this patient's condition?
   A) He will have an extremely friendly personality
   B) He may exhibit a positive Chvostek sign
   C) The diagnosis is confirmed with a western blot
   D) The condition is due to aberrant development of the 1st and 2nd pharyngeal pouches
   - **Correct answer is B**
   - **Cleft lip and palate, a cardiac murmur, and hypertelorism → DiGeorge syndrome (due to aberrant development of the 3rd and 4th pharyngeal pouches and can result in hypoparathyroidism)**
   - **↓ parathyroid → ↓ Ca^{2+} → positive Chvostek sign**

Section XII.1 - Cri-du-chat

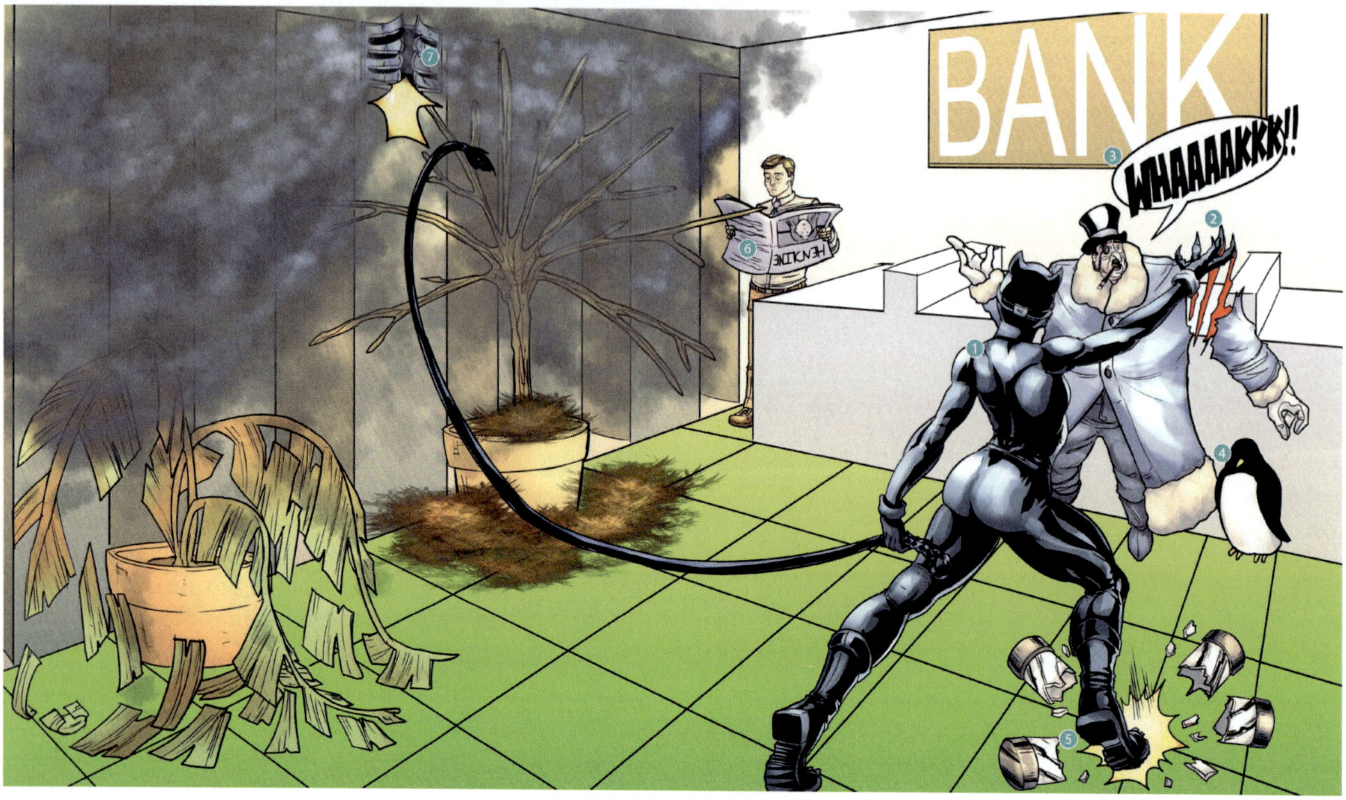

1. ______________________________
2. ______________________________
3. ______________________________
4. ______________________________
5. ______________________________
6. ______________________________
7. ______________________________

Section XII.2 - Williams Syndrome

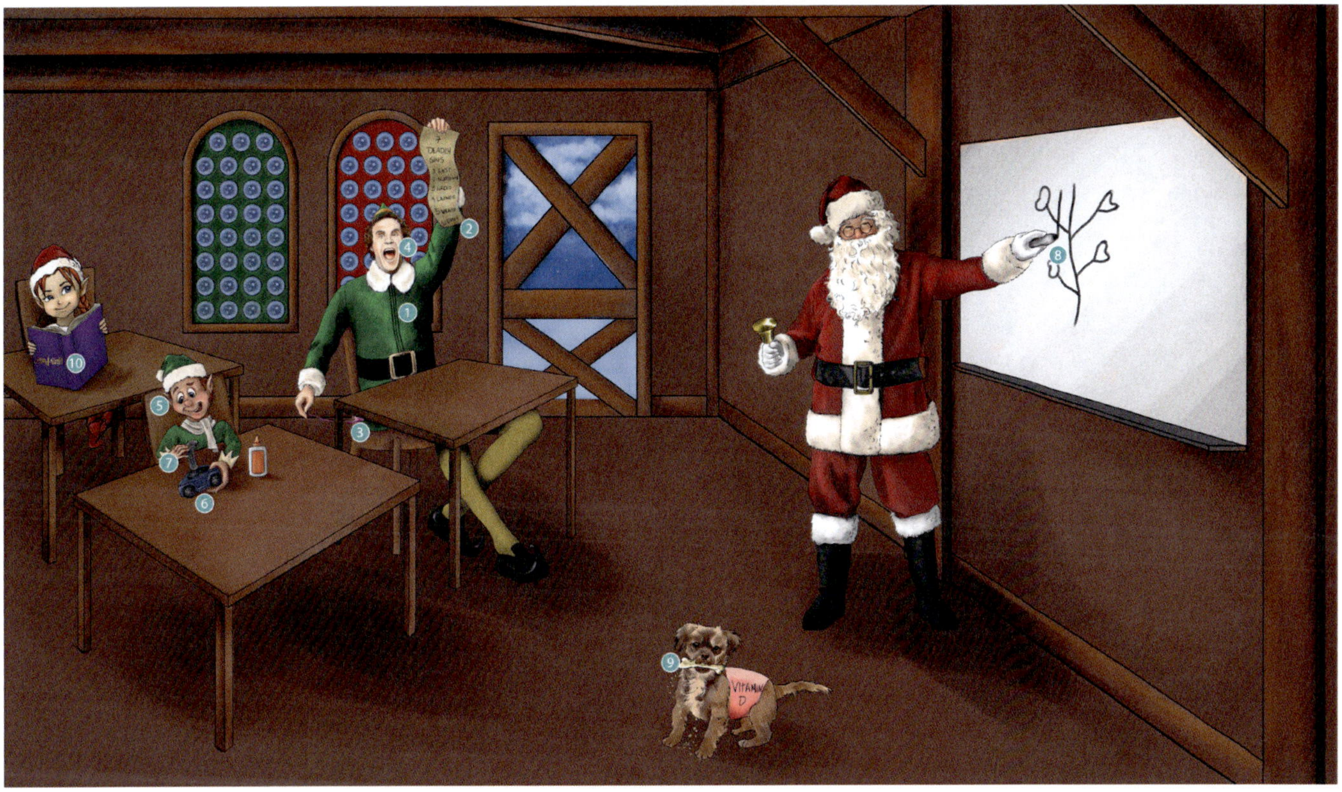

1. ____________________

2. ____________________

3. ____________________

4. ____________________

5. ____________________

6. ____________________

7. ____________________

8. ____________________

9. ____________________

10. ____________________

Section XII.3 - DiGeorge Syndrome

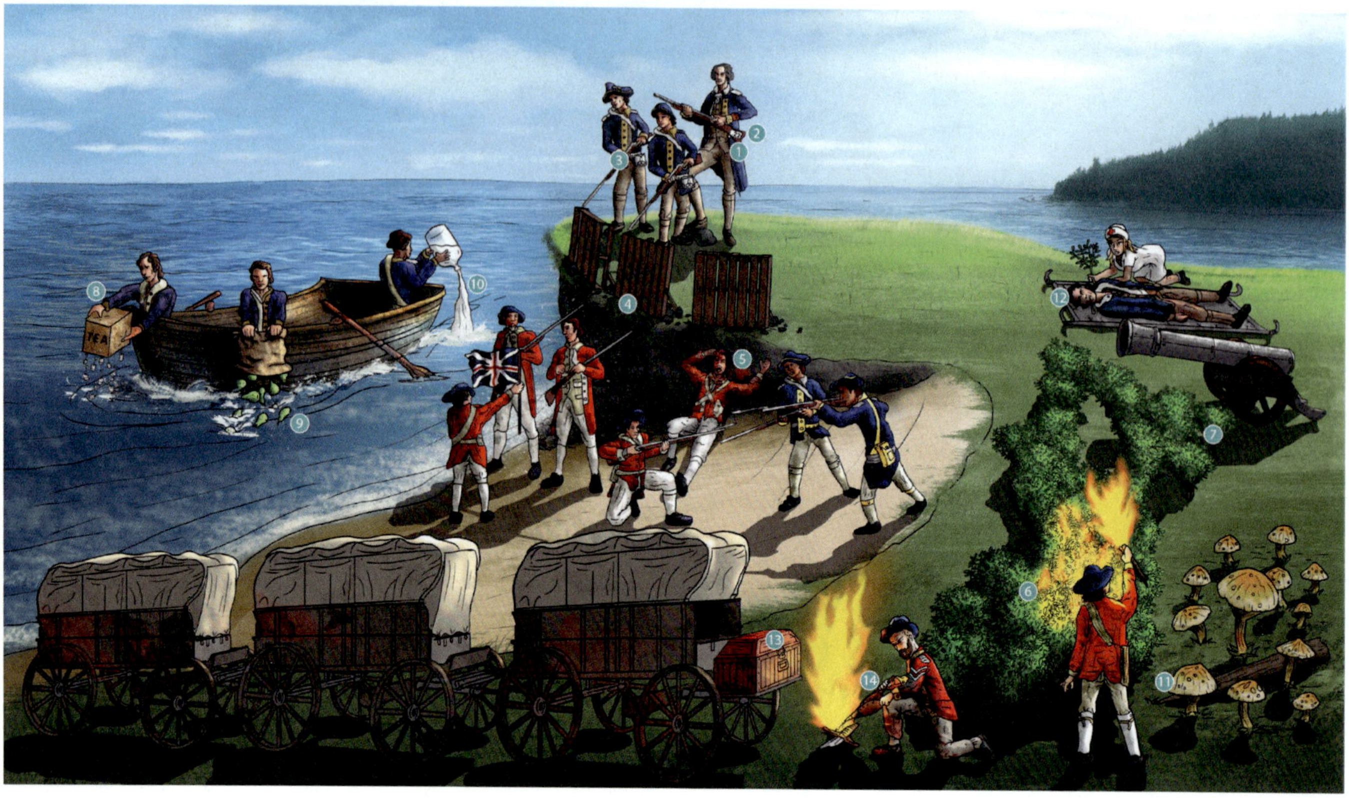

1. ______________________
2. ______________________
3. ______________________
4. ______________________
5. ______________________
6. ______________________
7. ______________________
8. ______________________
9. ______________________
10. ______________________
11. ______________________
12. ______________________
13. ______________________
14. ______________________

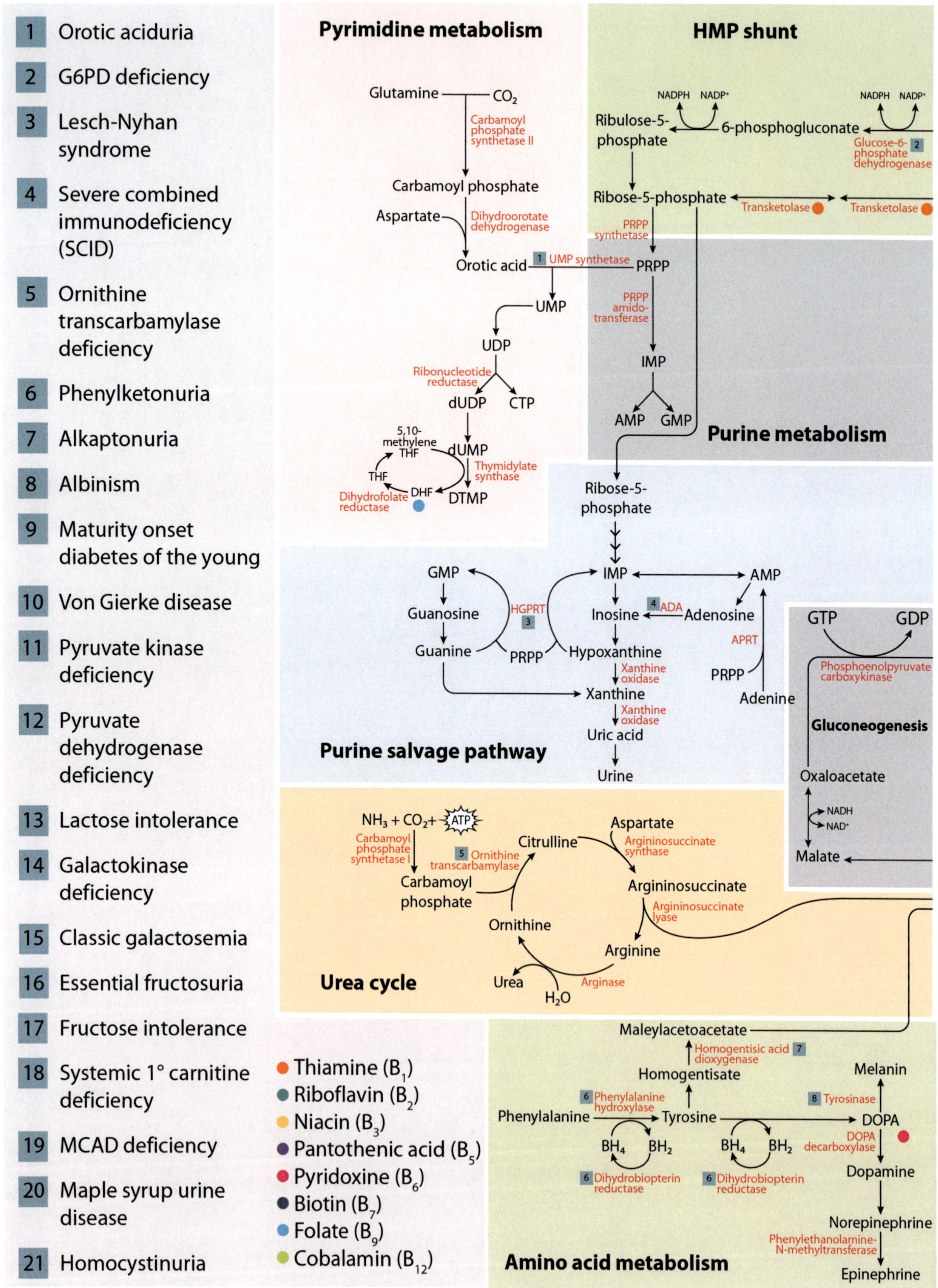

Figure 2.5.1 - Biochemistry map

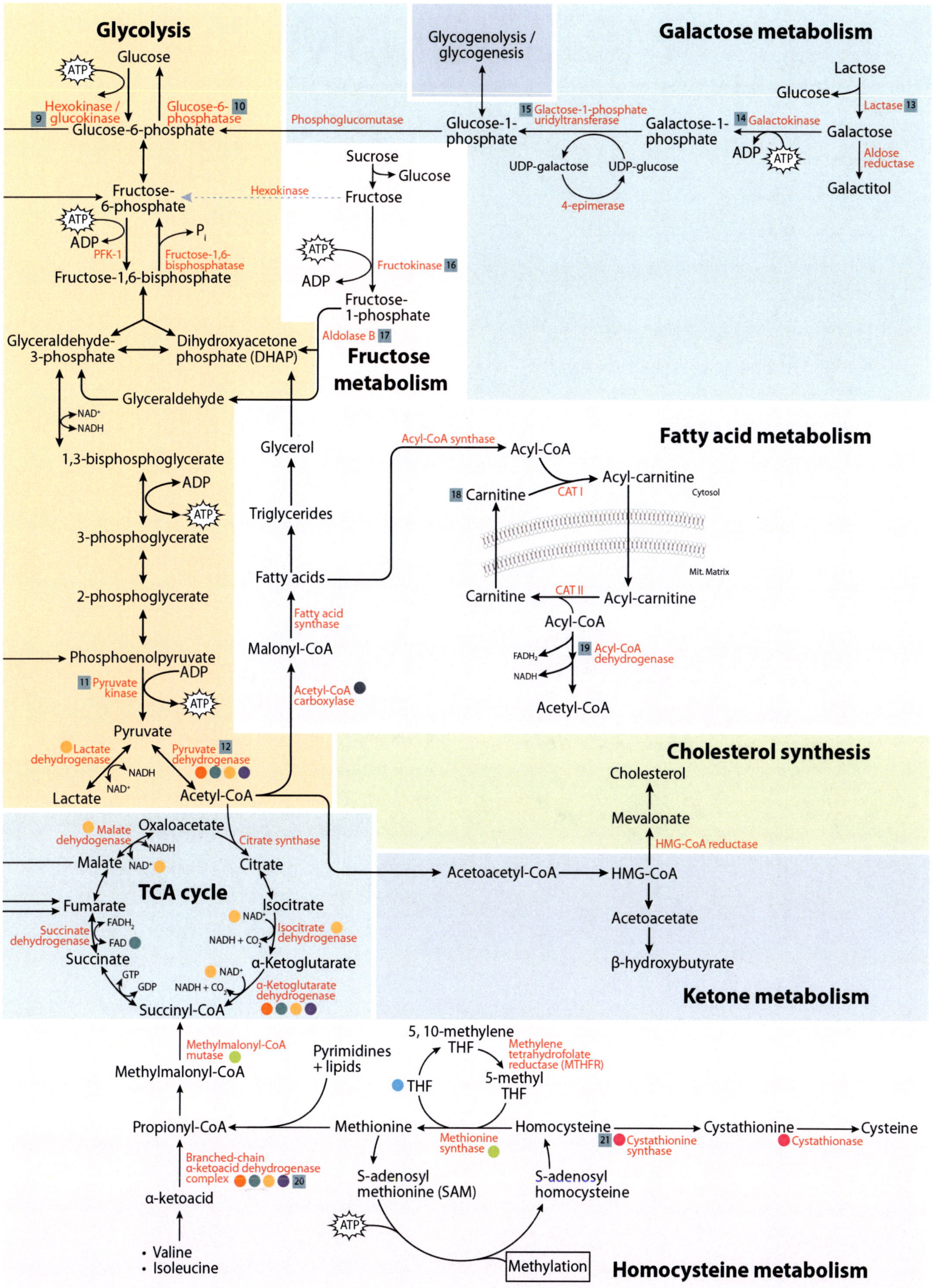

Glycolysis
Glucose
ATP
Hexokinase / glucokinase
9
Glucose-6- phosphatase
10
Glucose-6-phosphate
Fructose-6-phosphate
ATP
ADP
PFK-1
P_i
Fructose-1,6-bisphosphatase
Fructose-1,6-bisphosphate
Glyceraldehyde-3-phosphate
Dihydroxyacetone phosphate (DHAP)
Glyceraldehyde
NAD^+
NADH
1,3-bisphosphoglycerate
ADP
ATP
3-phosphoglycerate
2-phosphoglycerate
Phosphoenolpyruvate
11 Pyruvate kinase
ADP
ATP
Pyruvate
Lactate dehydrogenase
NADH
NAD^+
Lactate
Pyruvate dehydrogenase 12
Acetyl-CoA
Glycogenolysis / glycogenesis
Galactose metabolism
Lactose
Glucose
Lactase 13
Galactose
14 Galactokinase
ADP
ATP
Aldose reductase
Galactitol
Galactose-1-phosphate
15 Glactose-1-phosphate uridyltransferase
UDP-galactose
UDP-glucose
4-epimerase
Glucose-1-phosphate
Phosphoglucomutase
Sucrose
Glucose
Fructose
Hexokinase
ATP
ADP
Fructokinase 16
Fructose-1-phosphate
Aldolase B 17
Fructose metabolism
Glycerol
Triglycerides
Fatty acids
Fatty acid synthase
Malonyl-CoA
Acetyl-CoA carboxylase
Fatty acid metabolism
Acyl-CoA synthase
Acyl-CoA
Acyl-carnitine
18 Carnitine
CAT I
Cytosol
Mit. Matrix
Carnitine
CAT II
Acyl-carnitine
Acyl-CoA
$FADH_2$
NADH
19 Acyl-CoA dehydrogenase
Acetyl-CoA
Cholesterol synthesis
Cholesterol
Mevalonate
HMG-CoA reductase
Acetoacetyl-CoA
HMG-CoA
Acetoacetate
β-hydroxybutyrate
Ketone metabolism
Oxaloacetate
Malate dehydogenase
NADH
NAD^+
Malate
Citrate synthase
Citrate
TCA cycle
Fumarate
$FADH_2$
Succinate dehydrogenase
FAD
Succinate
Isocitrate
NAD^+
$NADH + CO_2$
Isocitrate dehydrogenase
α-Ketoglutarate
NAD^+
$NADH + CO_2$
α-Ketoglutarate dehydrogenase
GTP
GDP
Succinyl-CoA
Methylmalonyl-CoA mutase
Methylmalonyl-CoA
Propionyl-CoA
Branched-chain α-ketoacid dehydrogenase complex
20
α-ketoacid
• Valine
• Isoleucine
Pyrimidines + lipids
5, 10-methylene THF
Methylene tetrahydrofolate reductase (MTHFR)
THF
5-methyl THF
Methionine
Methionine synthase
Homocysteine
21 Cystathionine synthase
Cystathionine
Cystathionase
Cysteine
S-adenosyl methionine (SAM)
S-adenosyl homocysteine
ATP
Methylation
Homocysteine metabolism

Section I - Hexokinase & Glucokinase

I. Enzyme terminology

A. Kinases add phosphate groups (usually from ATP).

B. Phosphatases remove phosphate groups.

C. Phosphorylases add inorganic phosphate (usually without ATP).

D. Dehydrogenases perform redox reactions.

E. Mutase rearranges a functional group within the molecule.

F. Hydroxylases add a hydroxyl group (-OH).

G. Carboxylases transfer CO_2 groups.

II. Michaelis-Menten kinetics (Figure 2.5.2)

A. V_{max} = maximum speed of a reaction

B. K_m = the concentration of a substrate which permits the enzyme to achieve half of V_{max}

C. ↓ Km = ↑ affinity of the substrate for the enzyme (only low concentrations of the substrate are necessary for the enzyme to bind)

D. ↑ Km = ↓ affinity of the substrate for the enzyme (high concentrations of the substrate are necessary for the enzyme to bind)

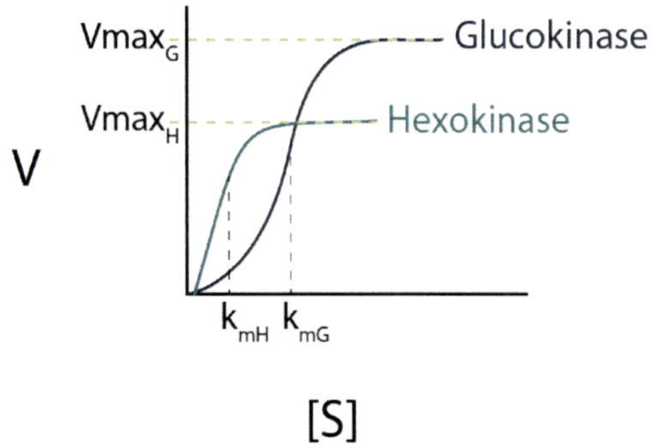

Figure 2.5.2 - Glucokinase and Hexokinase curves

III. Hexokinase

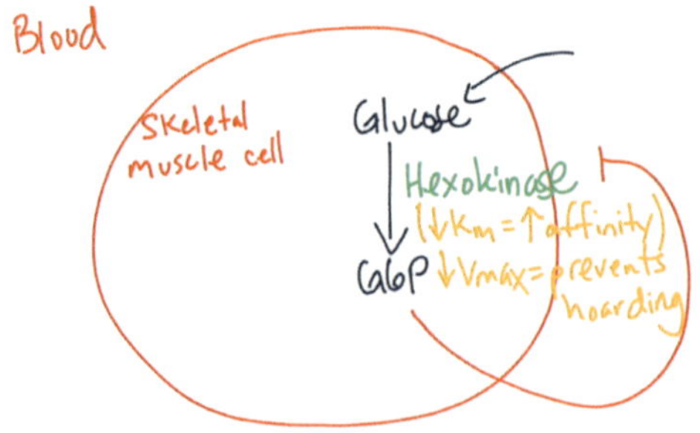

A. Present in most tissues (except pancreatic beta cells and liver)

B. Inhibited by glucose-6-phosphate

C. Not induced by insulin

D. ↓ Km → When glucose is present, the cell rapidly converts it into glucose-6-P → energy

E. ↓ Vmax → Prevents the cell from hoarding too much glucose and thus only utilizes what is needed

IV. Glucokinase

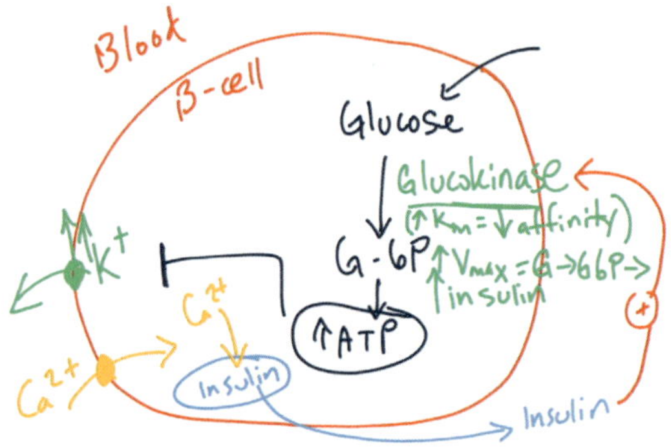

A. Present in pancreatic beta cells and liver

B. Not inhibited by glucose-6-phosphate

C. Induced by insulin

D. ↑ Km → ↓ glucose utilization by the liver when blood glucose concentrations are low

E. ↑ Vmax → ↑ ability of the liver to convert glucose → glycogen during well fed states

REVIEW QUESTIONS

1. An experiment is conducted to determine the maximum velocity of two enzymes. The results of the experiment are shown below.

Glucose concentration (mM)	Rate with enzyme X (µmol/L/sec)	Rate with enzyme Y (µmol/L/sec)
10	120	50
20	330	250
30	400	500
40	400	600
50	400	600

What enzyme from the experiment most closely resembles an enzyme in the glycolytic pathway that is regulated by concentrations of glucose-6-phosphate?

- **Vmax of enzyme X = 400 µmol/L/sec (substrate concentration of 30 mM)**
- **Vmax of enzyme Y = 600 µmol/L/sec (substrate concentration of 40 mM)**
- **The Vmax of enzyme X is reached at a lower substrate concentration than enzyme Y → has a lower Km than enzyme Y**
- **Enzyme X has a lower Km and Vmax than enzyme Y → it more closely resembles hexokinase (this is regulated by glucose-6-phosphate and glucokinase is not)**

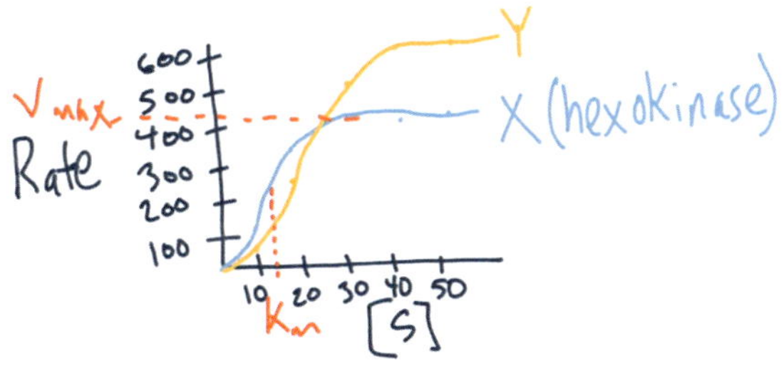

Section II - Glycolysis

I. Glycolysis overview (Figure 2.5.3)

A. A key metabolic pathway present in all cells that converts glucose to pyruvate

B. Occurs within the cytoplasm

C. Generates adenosine triphosphate (ATP) and nicotinamide adenine dinucleotide (NADH) → cellular energy

II. Regulation by fructose-2,6-bisphosphate

A. Fructose-2,6-bisphosphate regulates gluconeogenesis and glycolysis by controlling phosphofructokinase-1 (PFK-1).

B. Fructose-2,6-bisphosphate → ↑ PFK-1 → ↑ glycolysis

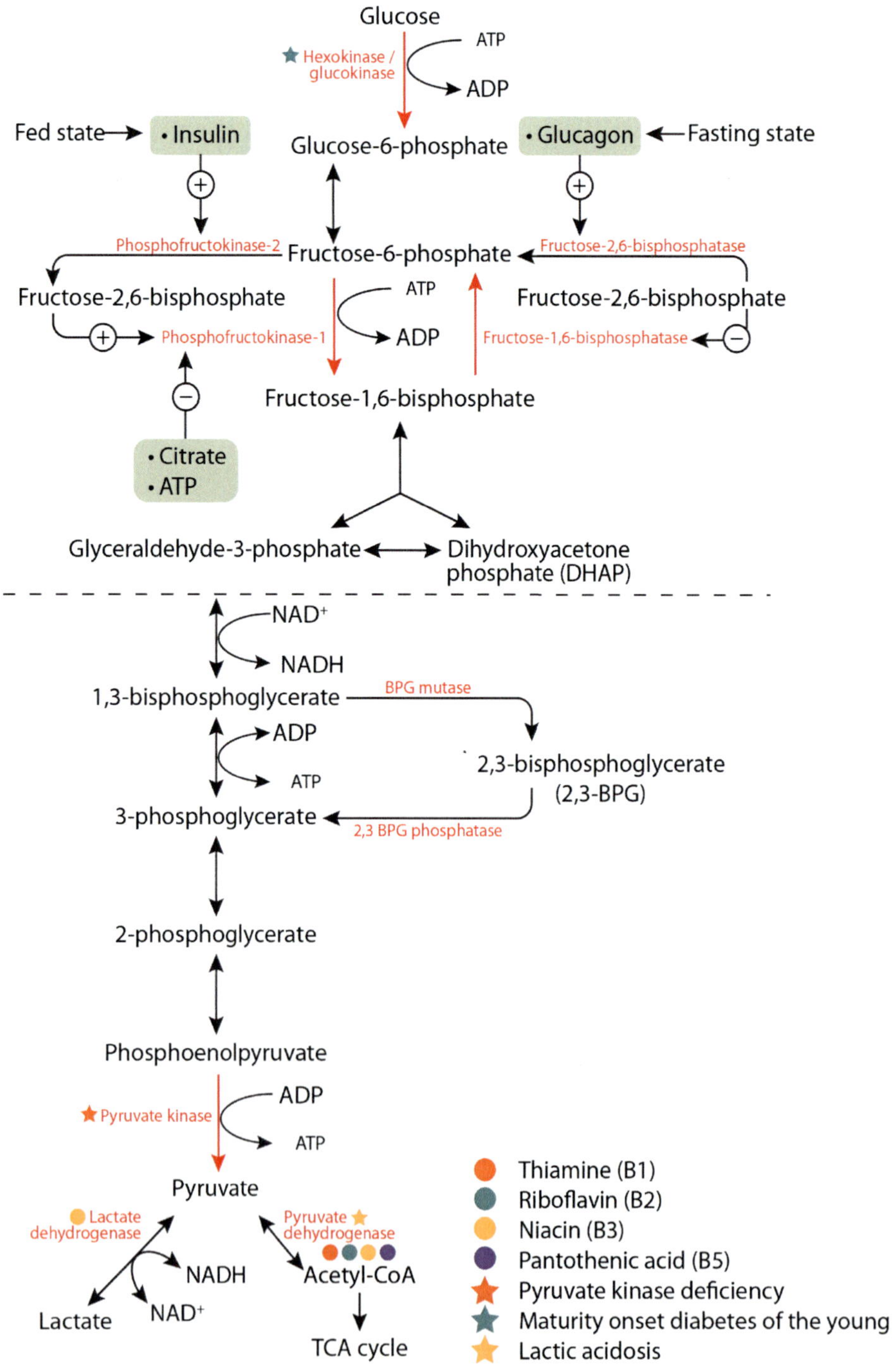

Figure 2.5.3 - Glycolysis

C. Fructose-2,6-bisphosphate → ↓ fructose-6-bisphosphatase → ↓ gluconeogenesis

D. Insulin (fed state) → ↑ fructose-2,6-bisphosphate → ↑ glycolysis and ↓ gluconeogenesis

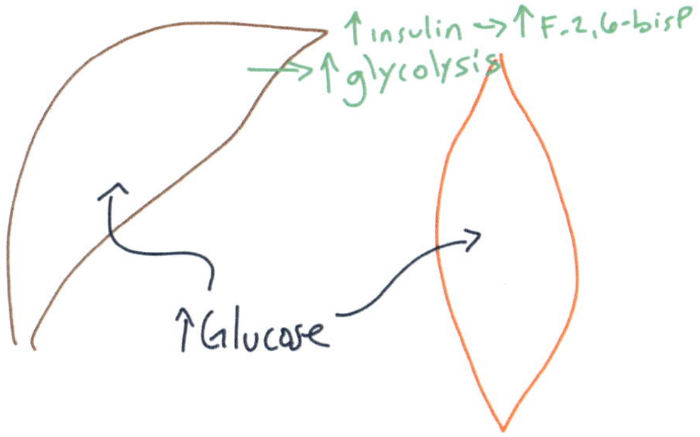

E. Glucagon (fasting state) → ↓ fructose 2,6-bisphosphate → ↓ glycolysis ↑ gluconeogenesis

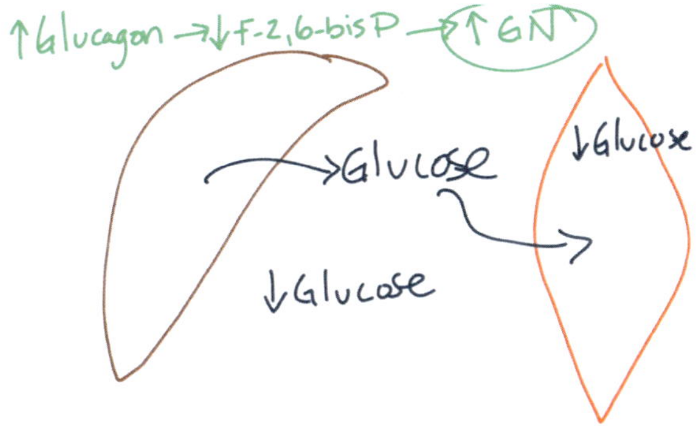

F. Citrate and ATP (represent a high intracellular energy state) → ↓ PFK-1 → ↓ glycolysis

III. 2,3-bisphosphoglycerate (2,3-BPG)

A. RBCs can bypass a step in glycolysis (1,3-BPG → 3-phosphoglycerate) in order to generate 2,3-BPG.

B. 2,3-BPG binds to hemoglobin → ↓ Hb affinity for O_2 → ↑ O_2 release into the peripheral tissues

C. This process sacrifices the production of ATP within RBCs.

IV. Pyruvate kinase

A. An enzyme that converts phosphoenolpyruvate (PEP) to pyruvate and generates ATP in the process.

B. Pyruvate kinase deficiency is an autosomal recessive disorder that is most pronounced in RBCs.

C. ↓ Pyruvate kinase → ↓ ATP → hemolysis

REVIEW QUESTIONS

1. A new drug is being studied by a pharmaceutical company. During a series of experiments the researchers notice that this drug decreases the hepatic concentration of fructose-2,6-bisphosphate. How will this drug likely alter the activity of aspartate transaminase (converts aspartate → oxaloacetate)?

- **↓ fructose-2,6-bisphosphate → ↑ gluconeogenesis → ↑ catabolism of amino acids → ↑ activity of aspartate transaminase (normally breaks down amino acids)**

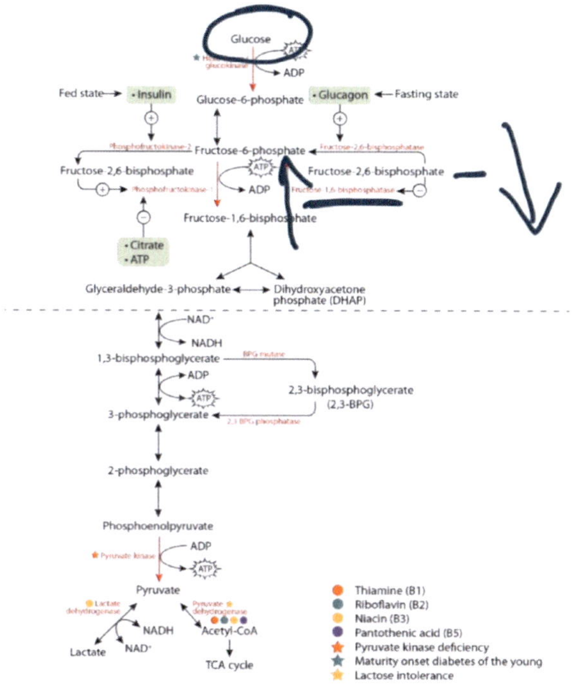

2. A 9-year-old boy presents to the physician for a routine visit. He has a history of anemia due to an enzyme deficiency. Physical exam reveals splenomegaly and conjunctival pallor. CBC shows an elevated reticulocyte count and confirms a hemolytic anemia. What mechanism explains this patient's anemia?

- **Pyruvate kinase normally converts PEP → pyruvate and generates ATP**
- **↓ pyruvate kinase → ↓ ATP → hemolysis**

Section III - Pyruvate Metabolism

I. Pyruvate can be converted into alanine, oxaloacetate, acetyl-CoA, and lactate. (Figure 2.5.4)

A. Pyruvate → alanine occurs primarily in muscle tissue during protein catabolism

B. Pyruvate → oxaloacetate is the first step in gluconeogenesis and occurs primarily in the liver

C. Pyruvate → acetyl-CoA occurs in many tissues under aerobic conditions

D. Pyruvate → lactate occurs in many tissues under anaerobic conditions

II. Pyruvate dehydrogenase complex

A. Requires 5 cofactors including thiamine (vitamin B_1), lipoic acid, CoA (vitamin B_5), FAD (vitamin B_2), and NAD (vitamin B_3).

B. Mnemonic: "TLC for Nancy."

III. Acetyl-CoA and NADH are key regulators of pyruvate metabolism.

A. Acetyl-CoA and NADH inhibit pyruvate dehydrogenase.

1. NADH is a product of the TCA cycle and is utilized in the electron transport chain (ETC).

2. Under hypoxic conditions the ETC is unable to utilize NADH resulting in elevations of NADH. This inhibits pyruvate dehydrogenase and signals the cell to shunt pyruvate to lactate.

3. In a well-fed state the TCA cycle is inhibited due to the accumulation of ATP (product of the ETC) and NADH → ↑ acetyl-CoA → ↑ inhibition of pyruvate dehydrogenase

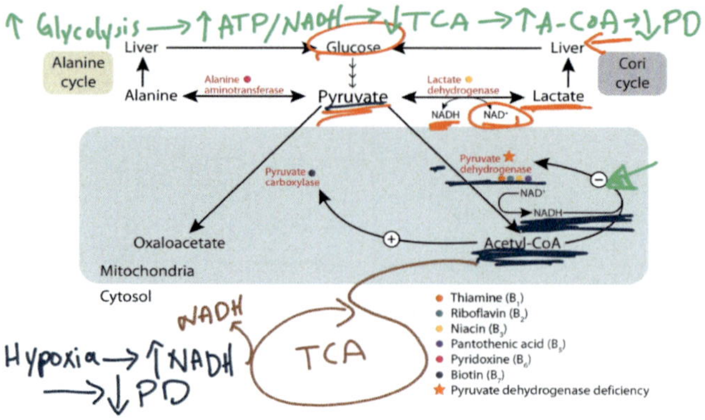

B. In liver tissue acetyl-CoA activates pyruvate carboxylase.

1. During periods of fasting, fatty acid metabolism increases → ↑ beta oxidation → ↑ acetyl-CoA → upregulation of pyruvate carboxylase

2. Thus acetyl-CoA increases gluconeogenesis and promotes the conversion glycerol, alanine, lactate, and other substances into pyruvate and then oxaloacetate.

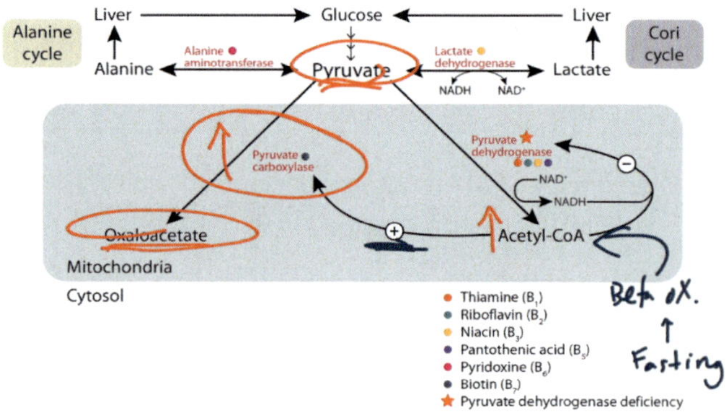

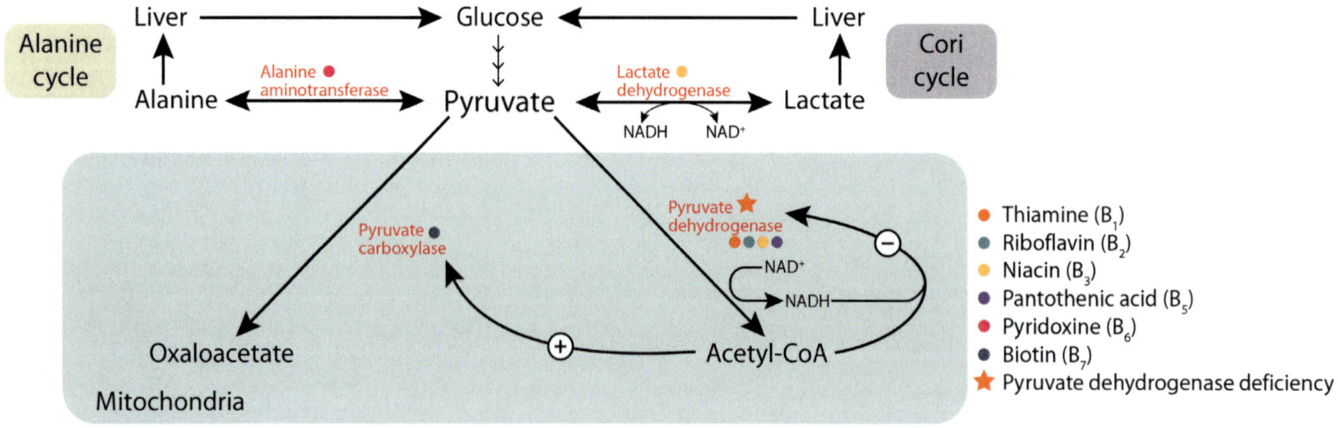

Figure 2.5.4 - Pyruvate metabolism

IV. Pyruvate dehydrogenase deficiency

A. An x-linked disorder resulting in reduced activity of pyruvate dehydrogenase → ↑ shunting of pyruvate to lactate and alanine → lactic acidosis

B. Dietary carbohydrates and amino acids are metabolized to pyruvate → worsening of lactic acidosis

C. Lysine and leucine are used as part of the treatment because these are ketogenic amino acids that bypass pyruvate and can be converted into acetyl-CoA → no rise in lactate

REVIEW QUESTIONS

1. Researchers are studying the regulation of glycolysis in skeletal muscle tissue during exercise in healthy mice (group A) and mice with a knockout mutation for lactate dehydrogenase (group B). They discover that the mice from group B have slower rates of glycolysis. What intermediate in the glycolytic pathway likely accumulates as a result of this mutation?

- **Lactate dehydrogenase normally generates NAD+ during the conversion of pyruvate → lactate**
- **Lactate dehydrogenase deficiency → ↑ NADH and ↓ NAD+**
- **In glycolysis the conversion of glyceraldehyde-3-phosphate → 1,3-bisphosphoglycerate requires NAD+**
- **↓ NAD+ → ↑ glyceraldehyde-3-phosphate**

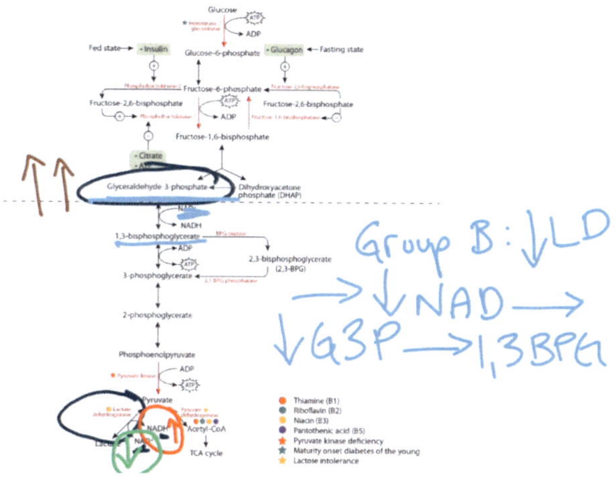

2. A 43-year-old male presents with a 30 minute history of severe substernal chest pain that radiates to his left arm. An EKG reveals ST segment elevations in leads II, III, and AVF. Several days after stabilization he is emergently transferred to the ICU in cardiogenic shock. How would the activity of pyruvate dehydrogenase and lactate dehydrogenase likely be altered in this patient?

- **In cardiogenic shock the tissues are not perfused adequately → ↓ O_2 → ↑ anaerobic metabolism → ↑ activity of lactate dehydrogenase**
- **Conversion of pyruvate to acetyl-CoA is not favored under hypoxic conditions → ↓ activity of pyruvate dehydrogenase**

Section IV - The Tricarboxylic Acid Cycle

I. Tricarboxylic acid (TCA) cycle overview (Figure 2.5.5)

A. A metabolic pathway that converts acetyl-CoA → CO_2

B. Generates NADH and $FADH_2$ → electron transport chain → cellular energy

1. Also generates guanosine triphosphate (GTP)

C. Occurs within the mitochondria.

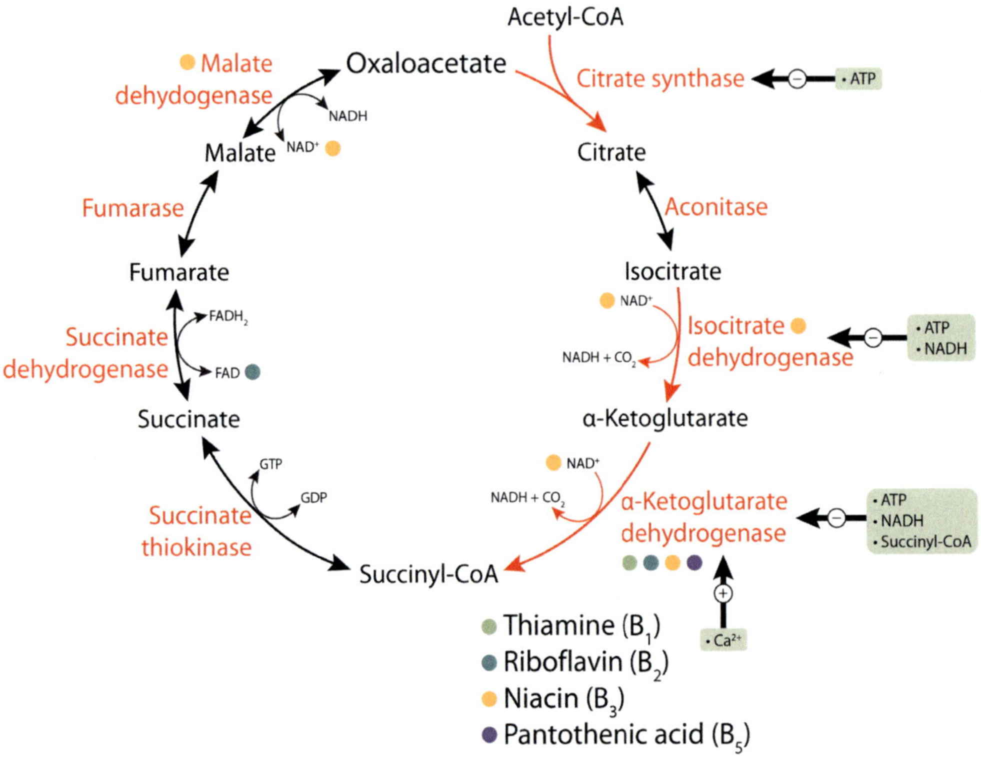

Figure 2.5.5 - TCA Cycle

II. Important enzymes

A. Citrate synthase

1. Oxaloacetate → citrate

a) Citrate is a marker of sufficient energy

b) Blocks phosphofructokinase-1 and decreases glycolysis

c) Activates acetyl-CoA carboxylase and increases fatty acid synthesis

2. Inhibited by ATP

B. Isocitrate dehydrogenase

1. Isocitrate → α-ketoglutarate dehydrogenase

2. Produces NADH and CO_2

3. Inhibited by ATP and NADH and activated by ADP

4. Requires niacin as a cofactor and for the production of NAD^+

C. α-ketoglutarate dehydrogenase

1. α-ketoglutarate → Succinyl-CoA

2. Produces NADH and CO_2

3. Inhibited by ATP, NADH, and Succinyl-CoA

4. Activated by Ca^{2+} in skeletal muscle tissue

5. Similar complex to pyruvate dehydrogenase

a) Requires 5 cofactors including thiamine (vitamin B_1), lipoic acid, CoA (vitamin B_5), FAD (vitamin B_2), and NAD (vitamin B_3).

b) Mnemonic: "TLC for Nancy."

D. Succinate thiokinase

1. Succinyl-CoA → succinate

2. Produces GTP

E. Succinate dehydrogenase

   1. Succinate → fumarate
   2. Complex II of the ETC
   3. FAD is a constituent of riboflavin (vitamin B_2) so this reaction is vitamin B_2-dependent.

F. Malate dehydrogenase

   1. Malate → oxaloacetate
   2. Niacin (Vitamin B_3) is necessary for the production of NAD^+ and acts as a cofactor for this enzyme.

REVIEW QUESTIONS ?

1. A 47-year-old homeless male is brought to the ED after being found unconscious on the side of the road. He is resuscitated and complains of difficulty walking and remembering past events. On exam he is ataxic and has ophthalmoplegia. What enzyme in the TCA cycle is likely altered as a result of this patient's condition?

   - **Memory loss, ataxia, and ophthalmoplegia are consistent with Wernicke-Korsakoff syndrome (caused by thiamine deficiency)**
   - **α-ketoglutarate is the only enzyme in the TCA cycle that requires thiamine as a cofactor**

2. A 24-year-old woman with a history of anorexia nervosa presents with fissures at the corners of her mouth and severe inflammation of her lips. On exam she has corneal clouding due to vascularization. What two reactions in the TCA cycle will likely be altered as a result of this patient's condition?

   - **Inflammation at the lips and fissures at the corners of her mouth → cheilosis**
   - **Cheilosis and corneal vascularization are seen in vitamin B_2 deficiency**
   - **↓ vitamin B_2 → ↓ α-ketoglutarate dehydrogenase (α-ketoglutarate → succinyl-CoA)**
   - **↓ vitamin B_2 → ↓ succinate dehydrogenase (succinate → fumarate)**

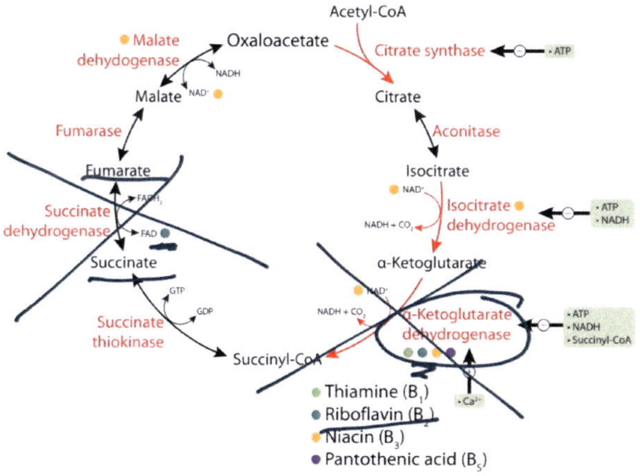

Section V - The Electron Transport Chain

I. Electron transport chain (ETC) overview

A. A group of complexes which utilize the energy from NADH and $FADH_2$ to produce ATP.

B. Occurs within the mitochondria.

C. The proteins used in the ETC are produced from the mitochondrial genome.

II. Phosphorylation

A. Oxidative phosphorylation: A process that generates ATP through ATP synthase as hydrogen ions move down their concentration gradient.

B. Substrate level phosphorylation: An enzymatic reaction that results in the formation of ATP via transfer of a phosphate group.

III. Oxidative phosphorylation

A. Energy from NADH and $FADH_2$ is transferred between molecules of the ETC, allowing the ETC to pump hydrogen ions from the mitochondrial matrix into the intermembrane space.

1. Electrons move from complex I → coenzyme Q → complex III → cytochrome C → complex IV

2. Complex II → coenzyme Q → complex III → cytochrome C → complex IV

B. Complex V (ATP synthase) synthesizes ATP as hydrogen ions move down their concentration gradient.

IV. Cytochromes

A. A class of proteins which contain heme groups.

B. Heme consists of a porphyrin ring with a center molecule of iron.

C. Hemoglobin in RBCs favors the Fe^{2+} state.

D. Iron in complex IV (cytochrome C oxidase) can vary between the Fe^{2+} and Fe^{3+} state.

V. Oxidative phosphorylation poisons

A. Rotenone blocks complex I.

B. Cyanide and carbon monoxide block complex IV.

1. Cyanide binds iron in the Fe^{3+} state (binds complex IV but not Hb in RBCs).

a) Amyl nitrite oxidizes hemoglobin in RBCs from Fe^{2+} to Fe^{3+} which can sequester cyanide in the blood.

2. Carbon monoxide has a high affinity for the Fe^{2+} state → disrupts Hb in RBCs and complex IV

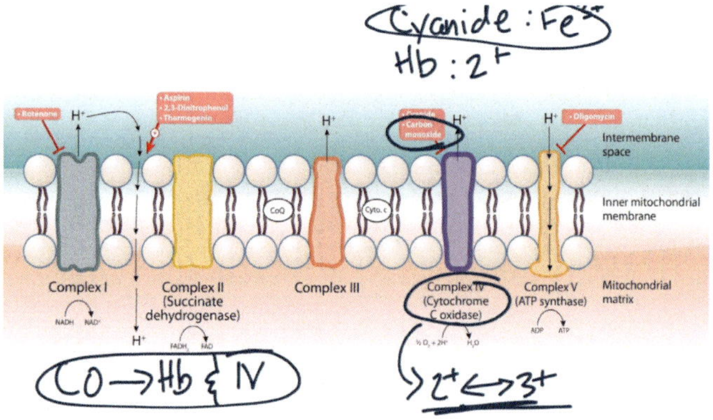

C. Oligomycin blocks ATP synthase.

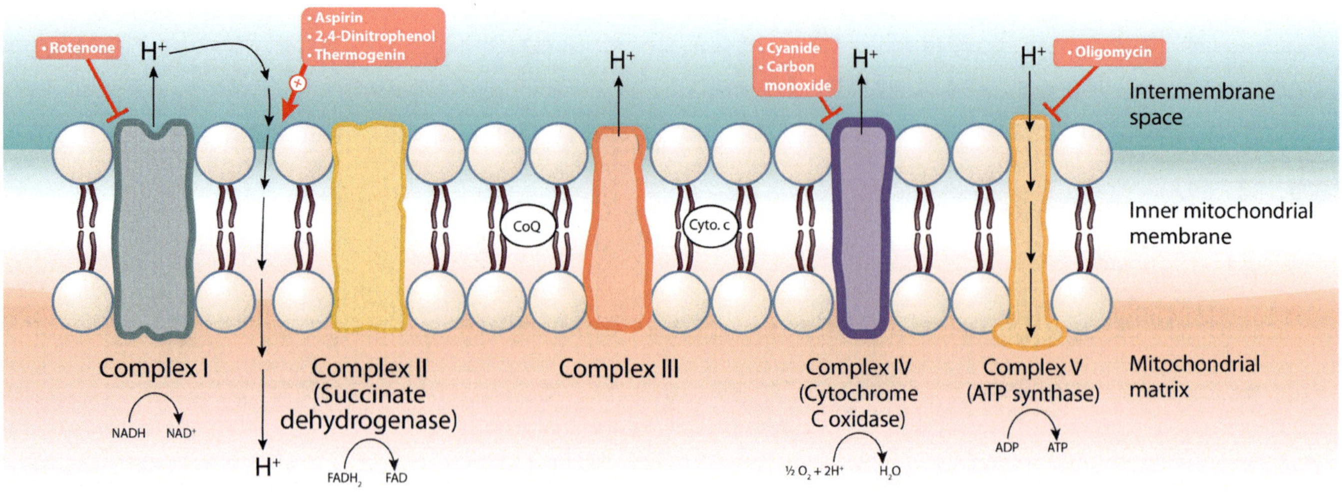

Figure 2.5.6 - ETC

REVIEW QUESTIONS

1. A 45-year-old male with a history of hypertension presents to the ED with a blood pressure of 190/123 and proteinuria. He is started on a medication used to control his blood pressure but then develops reddish skin discoloration and a severe headache. Repeat labs reveals a lactic acidosis. This patient's symptoms are most likely due to a substance which has a high affinity for what compound?

- **Reddish skin discoloration and headache → cyanide poisoning**
- **Nitroprusside is used to treat hypertensive emergency and contains cyanide side groups in its molecular structure (can cause cyanide poisoning)**
- **Cyanide preferentially binds Fe^{3+} → inhibition of complex IV → lactic acidosis**

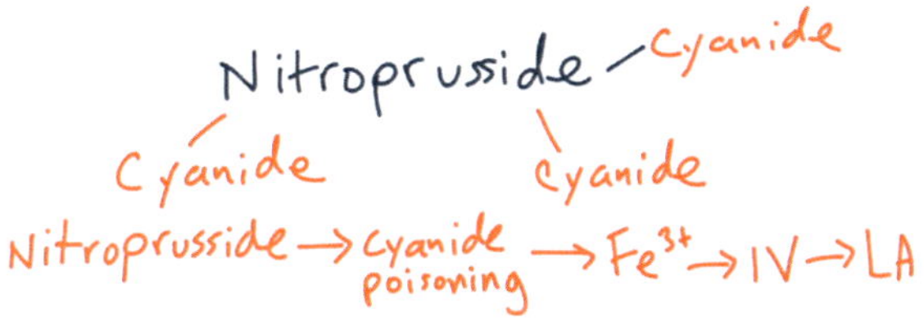

2. The patient is treated with a compound that results in resolution of his symptoms. However, while drawing blood for repeat labs, his blood now appears brown. What is the mechanism which explains the discoloration of the blood?

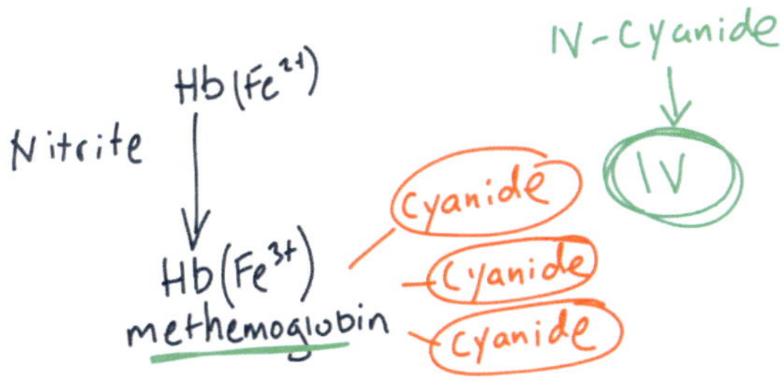

- **The treatment for cyanide poisoning is nitrite**
- **Nitrite oxidizes hemoglobin from the Fe^{2+} state → Fe^{3+} state (methemoglobin)**
- **Cyanide has a high affinity for the Fe^{3+} state, thus allowing methemoglobin to bind cyanide and liberate it from complex IV of the ETC → continuation of aerobic metabolism**
- **The brown colored blood is caused by methemoglobin**

Section VI - Gluconeogenesis

I. Gluconeogenesis overview (Figure 2.5.7)

A. A metabolic pathway that uses non-carbohydrates to produce glucose.

1. Non-carbohydrates include lactate, amino acids, glycerol, and propionyl-CoA (odd-chain fatty acids).

B. Occurs in the liver and kidneys.

C. An important pathway responsible for maintaining blood glucose levels.

B. Phosphoenolpyruvate carboxykinase

1. Oxaloacetate → PEP

2. Requires GTP (produced from the TCA cycle)

C. Fructose-1,6-bisphosphatase

1. Fructose-1,6-bisphosphate → fructose-6-phosphate

2. Tightly regulated by the concentration of fructose-2,6-bisphosphate

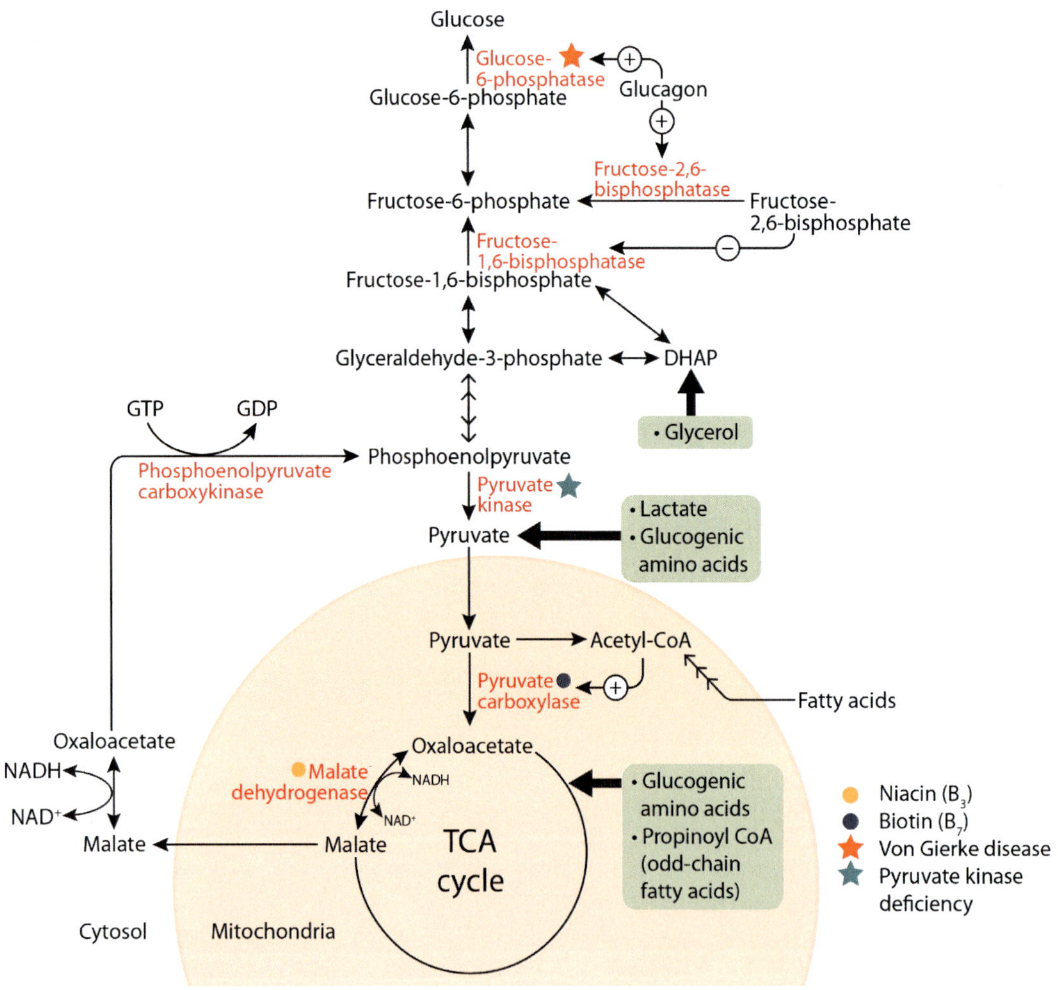

Figure 2.5.7 - Gluconeogenesis

II. Important enzymes

A. Pyruvate carboxylase

1. Pyruvate → oxaloacetate

2. Acetyl-CoA increases the activity of this enzyme.

a) Fatty acid metabolism → ↑ acetyl-CoA

b) ATP produced by the ETC → inhibition of the TCA cycle → ↑ acetyl-CoA

3. Requires vitamin B_7 (biotin)

3. Glucagon → ↓ fructose-2,6-bisphosphate → ↑ activity of fructose-1,6-bisphosphatase → ↑ gluconeogenesis

D. Glucose-6-phosphatase

E. Glucose-6-phosphate → glucose

1. Glucagon increases the activity of this enzyme.

REVIEW QUESTIONS

1. An experiment is performed on mice which have a knockout mutation resulting in an inability to metabolize triglycerides. The mice are deprived of food but given plenty of water. After several days without food the activity of several enzymes are analyzed. How will the activity of the enzymes pyruvate carboxylase and glycerol kinase likely be altered in the knockout mice compared to healthy mice?

- **↓ triglyceride metabolism → ↓ fatty acid oxidation → ↓ acetyl-CoA → ↓ pyruvate carboxylase → ↓ gluconeogenesis**
- **↓ triglyceride metabolism → ↓ glycerol → ↓ glycerol kinase**

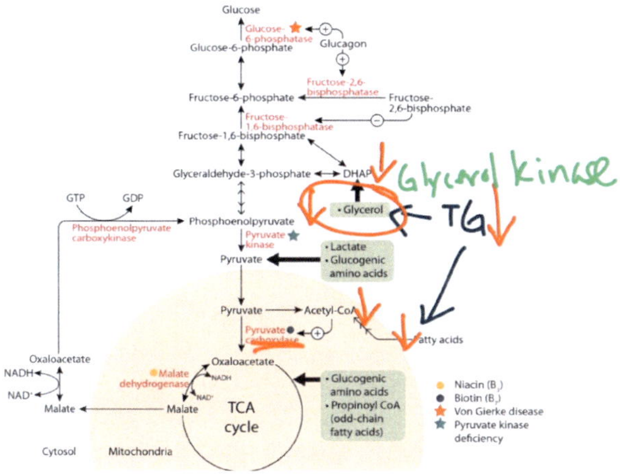

2. A 17-year-old male presents with a 2 month history of weight loss, depression and a rest blistering rash primarily affecting the legs. Two days ago he developed a DVT. On physical exam he has a rash consistent with necrolytic migratory erythema. Labs reveal hyperglycemia. How will the activity of fructose-1,6-bisphosphatase and glucose-6-phosphatase likely be altered in this patient?

- **Dermatitis, depression, declining weight, diabetes, and DVTs → glucagonoma**
- **Glucagon decreases the concentration of fructose-2,6-bisphosphate → ↑ activity of fructose-1,6-bisphosphatase**
- **Glucagon increases the activity of glucose-6-phosphatase → ↑ blood glucose (hyperglycemia)**

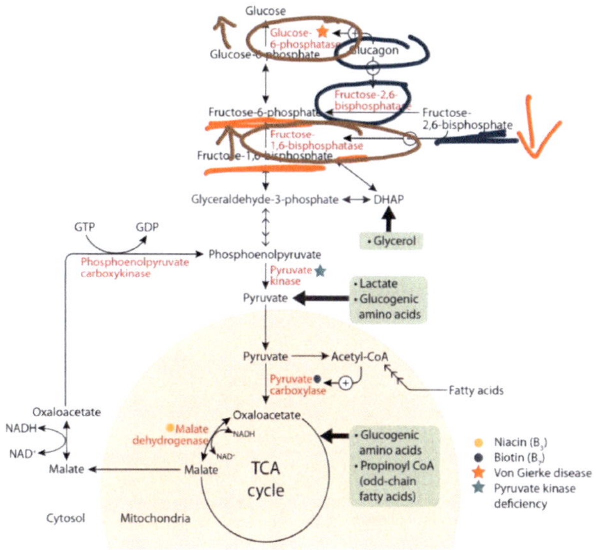

Section VII - Glycogen

I. Glycogen overview (Figure 2.5.8 - Glycogen metabolism)

A. A complex polymer of glucose that is stored in liver and muscle tissue.

B. Can be synthesized (glycogenesis) during periods of rest, or catabolized (glycogenolysis) for immediate energetic needs.

C. Linkages are formed by α-(1,4) bonds and branches are formed by α-(1,6) bonds.

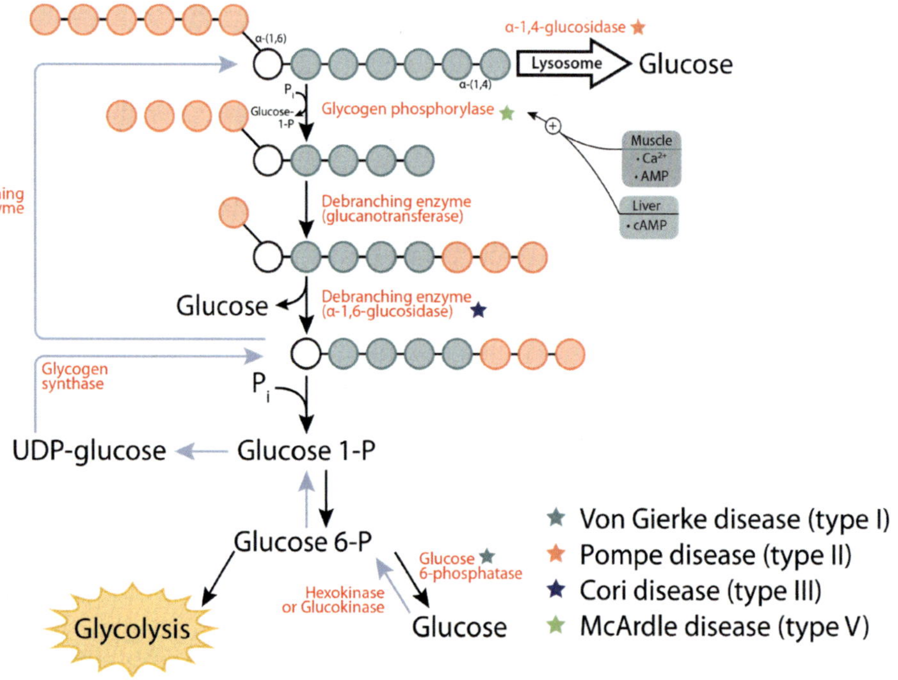

Figure 2.5.8 - Glycogen metabolism

II. Glycogen storage diseases (Table 2.5.1)

Disease	Enzyme	Findings	Mnemonics
Von Gierke disease (type I)	Glucose-6-phosphatase	• Liver cannot release glucose into blood → hypoglycemia • Accumulation of hepatic glycogen → hepatomegaly • Cori cycle defective → lactic acidosis	"Gierke breaks Gluconeogenesis"
Pompe disease (type II)	α-1,4-glucosidase (acid α-glucosidase)	• Lysosomal accumulation of glycogen in liver and muscle → cardiomegaly, hepatomegaly, and hypotonia. • Gluconeogenesis and glycogenolysis mostly normal → normal blood glucose levels	"PomPe breaks the PumP"
Cori disease (type III)	α-1,6-glucosidase	• Glycogen accumulation → hepatomegaly and hypotonia • ↓ glycogen mobilization → hypoglycemia → ↑ compensation via gluconeogenesis (i.e. fat metabolism) → ketoacidosis	"Cori breaks the Corner"
McArdle disease (type V)	Glycogen phosphorylase (only skeletal Muscle)	• ↓ glycogen breakdown → ↓ ATP → muscle cramps, muscle weakness, exercise intolerance, and rhabdomyolysis • Liver unaffected → normal blood glucose levels	"McArdle breaks the Muscle"

Table 2.5.1 - Glycogen storage diseases

A. Pompe disease (type II)

1. Caused by a deficiency of the enzyme acid α-1,4-glucosidase (acid α-glucosidase).
2. Normally breaks down glycogen within lysosomes in tissues where glycogen content is high (i.e. liver and muscle tissue).
3. Lysosomal accumulation of glycogen within liver and muscle tissue → cardiomegaly, hepatomegaly, and hypotonia
4. Gluconeogenesis and glycogenolysis mostly intact → normal blood glucose levels

B. McArdle disease (type V)

1. Deficiency of glycogen phosphorylase enzyme present in skeletal muscle tissue.
2. Activity increased by Ca^{2+} and AMP in muscle tissue and cAMP in liver tissue.
3. ↓ glycogen breakdown in skeletal muscle tissue → ↓ ATP → muscle cramps, muscle weakness, exercise intolerance, and rhabdomyolysis
4. Liver is unaffected → normal blood glucose levels

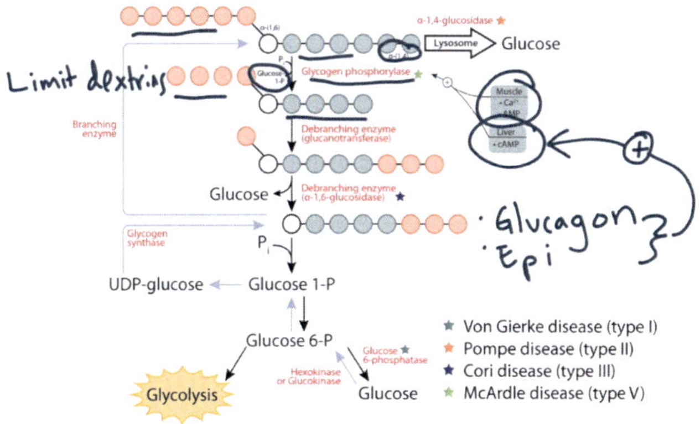

C. Cori disease (type III)

1. Caused by a debranching enzyme deficiency (α-1,6-glucosidase).
   a) Glucosyltransferase cleaves and transfers 3 of the 4 outer glucose residues.
   b) α-1,6-glucosidase removes the final branched glucose residue.
2. Clinical features include hypotonia, hepatomegaly, and hypoglycemia.
3. ↓ glycogen mobilization → ↑ compensation via gluconeogenesis (i.e. fat metabolism) → ketoacidosis

D. Von Gierke Disease (type I)

1. Deficiency of glucose-6-phosphatase → liver cannot get glucose out into the blood → hypoglycemia
2. Accumulation of hepatic glycogen → hepatomegaly
3. Cori cycle cannot recycle lactate → lactic acidosis

REVIEW QUESTIONS

1. A 6-month-old girl presents with developmental delay. Physical exam is significant for hepatomegaly and hypotonia. Her blood glucose level is normal. An EKG is significant for giant QRS complexes in all leads. A glycogen storage disease is suspected. What enzyme is most likely deficient?

- **The QRS complex represents ventricular depolarization**
- **Giant QRS complexes → large ventricles (cardiomegaly)**
- **Pompe disease is the only glycogen storage disease (type II) that causes cardiomegaly**
- **Pompe disease is caused by a deficiency of α-1,4-glucosidase**

2. A 2-year-old boy presents with growth failure and skeletal muscle wasting after a syncopal episode. Physical exam is significant for hepatomegaly. Labs reveal hypoglycemia and a mild ketoacidosis. A muscle biopsy reveals enlarged cells containing periodic acid-Schiff (PAS)-positive material. The enzyme that is most likely deficient performs what important function?

- **Hepatomegaly, hypoglycemia, and a mild ketoacidosis → Cori disease (glycogen storage disease type III)**
- **Cori disease is caused by a deficiency of α-1,6-glucosidase**
- **This enzyme removes the final branched glucose residue in glycogen**

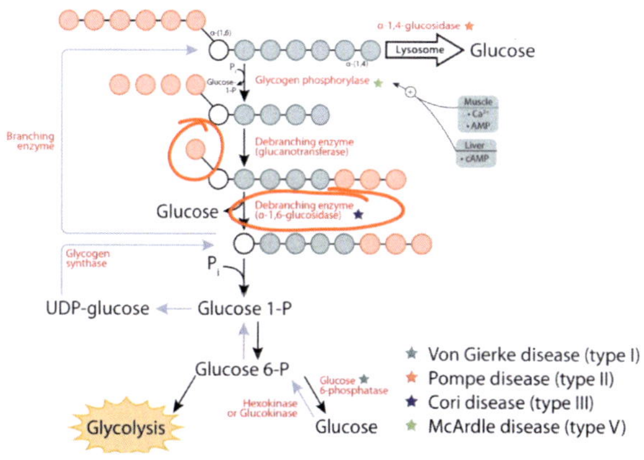

Section VII.1 - Von Gierke & Cori

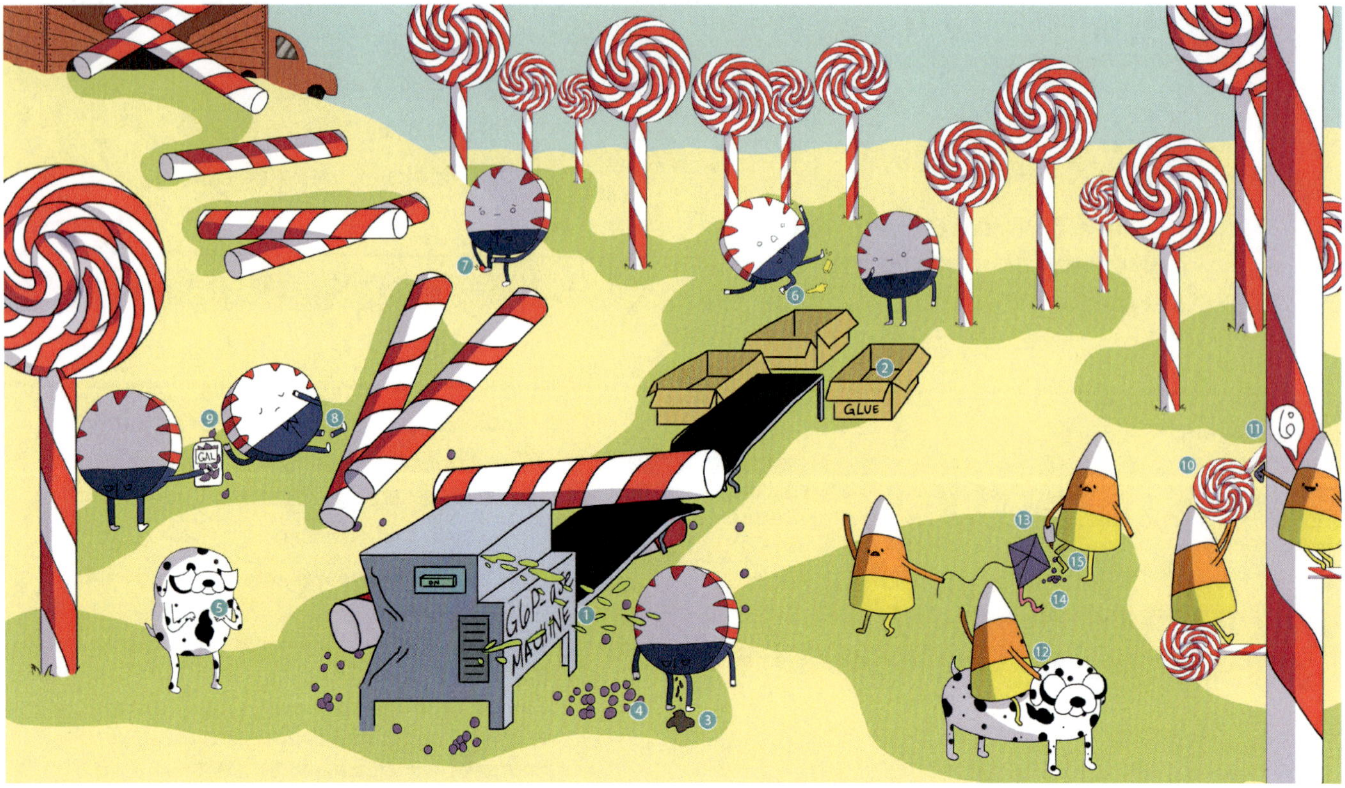

1. ______________________
2. ______________________
3. ______________________
4. ______________________
5. ______________________
6. ______________________
7. ______________________
8. ______________________
9. ______________________
10. ______________________
11. ______________________
12. ______________________
13. ______________________
14. ______________________
15. ______________________

Section VII.2 - Pompe & Mcardle

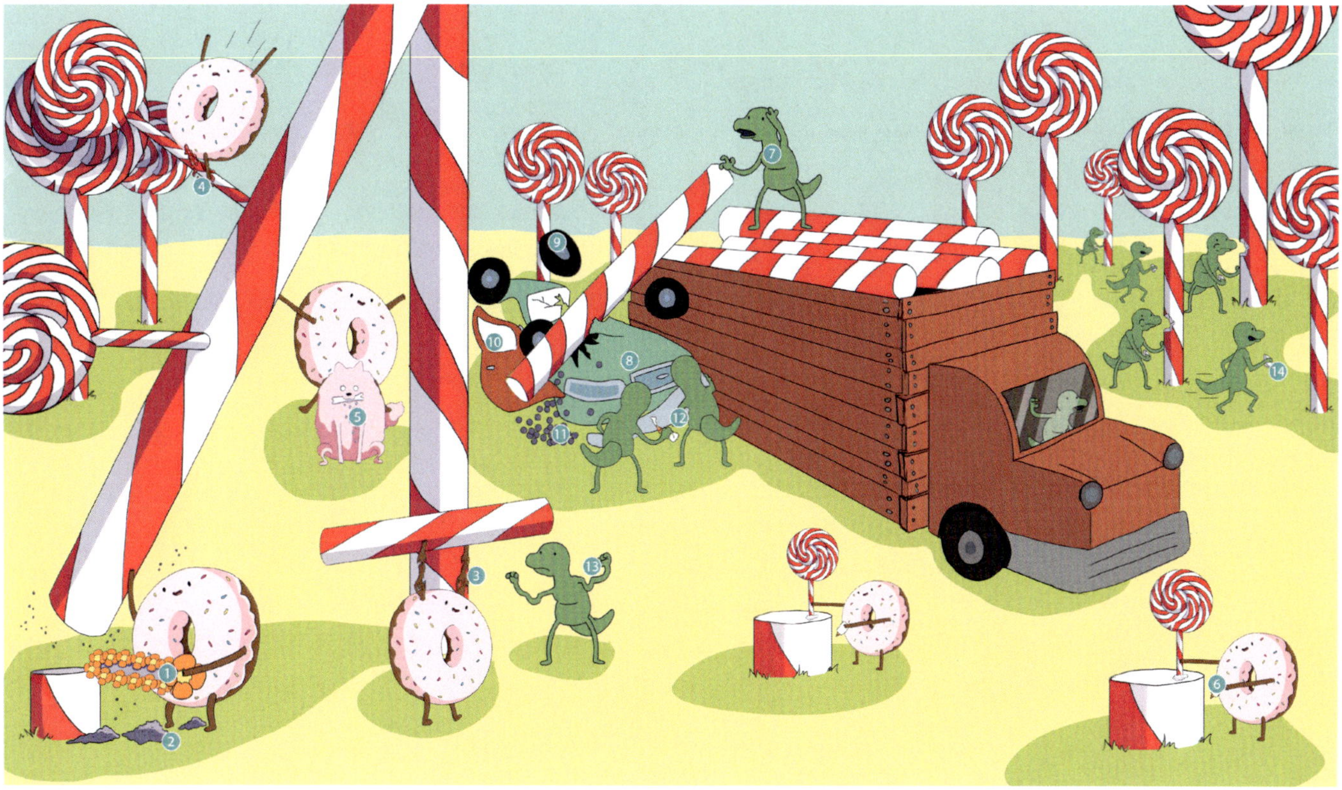

1. ______________________

2. ______________________

3. ______________________

4. ______________________

5. ______________________

6. ______________________

7. ______________________

8. ______________________

9. ______________________

10. ______________________

11. ______________________

12. ______________________

13. ______________________

14. ______________________

Section VIII - Fructose

I. Essential fructosuria (Figure 2.5.9)

A. Caused by a deficiency of the enzyme fructokinase.

B. Patients maintain the ability to metabolize some fructose due to compensatory pathways → asymptomatic

C. Can be detected in the urine by a copper reduction test (a nonspecific test that detects the presence of any reducing sugar [i.e. galactose, glucose, fructose, ribose, etc.]).

II. Fructose intolerance

A. Caused by a deficiency of the enzyme aldolase B.

B. ATP depletion in hepatocytes → inhibition of gluconeogenesis and glycogenolysis → hypoglycemia

C. Accumulation of metabolites in the liver → hepatomegaly

D. Can be detected in the urine by a copper reduction test (a nonspecific test that detects the presence of any reducing sugar [i.e. galactose, glucose, fructose, ribose, etc.]).

E. Symptoms occur following digestion of sucrose or other compounds containing fructose (fruit, honey, etc.).

III. Polyol pathway (Figure 2.5.10)

A. A metabolic pathway responsible for the conversion of glucose into fructose.

B. This pathway results in the production of sorbitol, which is an important contributor to the pathophysiology of cataracts.

1. Under the conditions of hyperglycemia, glucose is quickly metabolized into sorbitol.
2. The rate of sorbitol formation is faster than the rate of its conversion into fructose.
3. Sorbitol is an osmotic agent → ↑ influx of water into cells → cellular damage
4. Hyperglycemia → ↑ sorbitol → osmotic damage → cataract formation

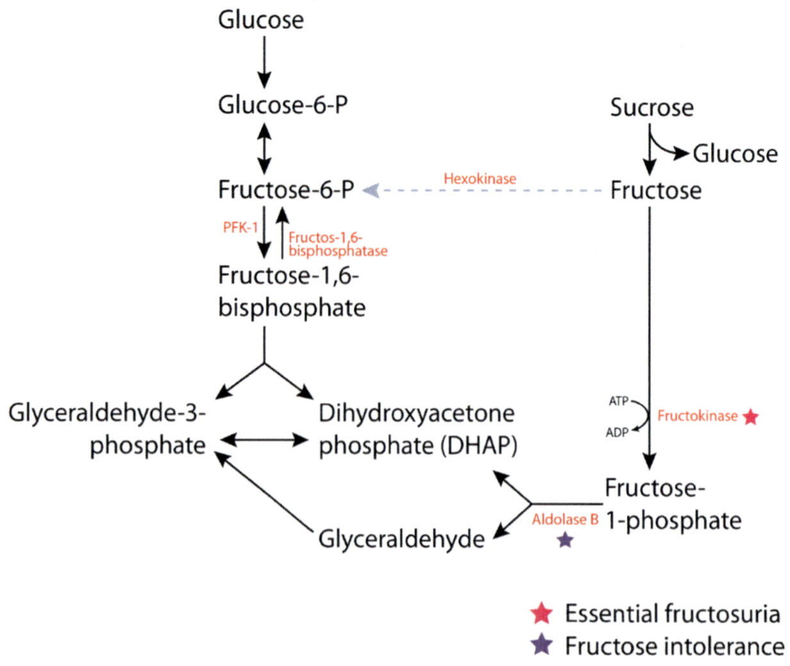

Figure 2.5.9 - Fructose metabolism

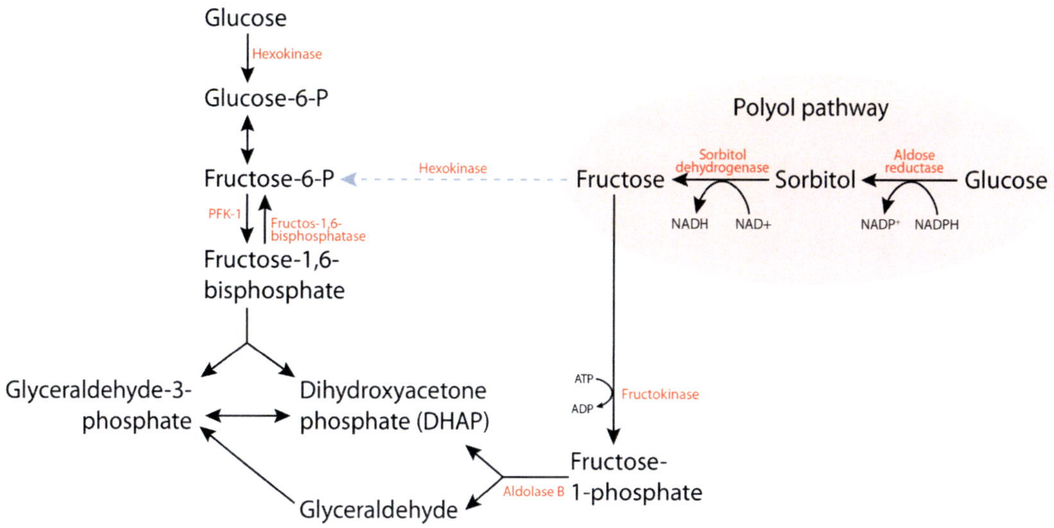

Figure 2.5.10 - Polyol pathway

REVIEW QUESTIONS

1. A previously healthy 8-month-old girl presents to the ED with nausea and vomiting. Her mother states that her symptoms started approximately 3 days ago. She also states that her daughter has been excessively tired. Labs reveal hypoglycemia. Her mother mentions that they recently began feeding her bottled food when her symptoms began. The most likely deficient enzyme in this patient results in hypoglycemia through what mechanism?
   - **Nausea, vomiting, and hypoglycemia after the introduction of bottled food → hereditary fructose intolerance (deficiency of aldolase B)**
   - **ATP is required to produce fructose-1-phosphate but it cannot be further metabolized → ATP depletion in hepatocytes → inhibition of gluconeogenesis and glycogenolysis → hypoglycemia**

2. An experiment is performed on two groups of mice. Mice from group A have a fructokinase deficiency and mice from group B are healthy. The mice are fed fructose and the rates of fructose metabolism are analyzed. How will the rate of fructose metabolism in mice from group A likely compare to that of mice from group B?
   - **Fructose can be metabolized directly into fructose-6-phosphate by the enzyme hexokinase in mice with a fructokinase deficiency (group A)**
   - **Fructose-6-phosphate is above the rate limiting step of glycolysis (phosphofructokinase-1) → slower rate of fructose metabolism**
   - **Mice from group B can metabolize fructose in the traditional pathway, thus bypassing PFK-1 → faster rate of fructose metabolism**

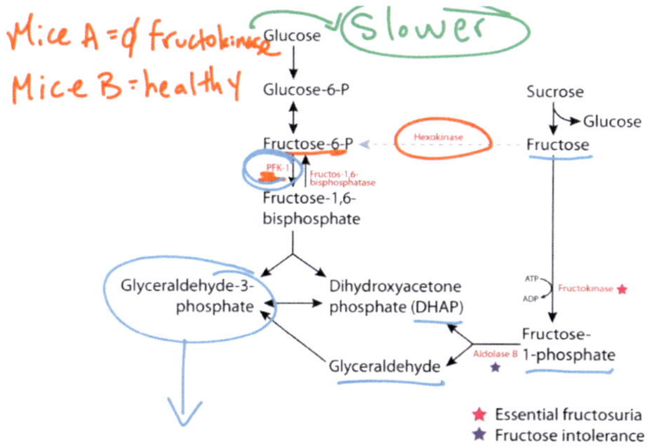

Section IX - Galactose

I. Lactase deficiency (Figure 2.5.11)

A. Symptoms include bloating, flatulence, and osmotic diarrhea that occurs after the digestion of lactose.

B. Primary lactose intolerance is caused by a genetic-related reduction of lactase production.

C. Secondary lactose intolerance is an acquired condition due to damage to the small intestine.

II. Galactokinase deficiency

A. Autosomal recessive hereditary deficiency of galactokinase.

B. ↑ galactose → ↑ shunting to galactitol → infantile cataracts

III. Classic galactosemia

A. Caused by a deficiency of galactose-1-phosphate uridyltransferase

B. Galactose-1-phosphate accumulates in cells → liver damage

C. ↑ Galactitol → cataracts

D. ATP depletion in hepatocytes → inhibition of gluconeogenesis and glycogenolysis → hypoglycemia

E. ↑ risk of e. coli sepsis.

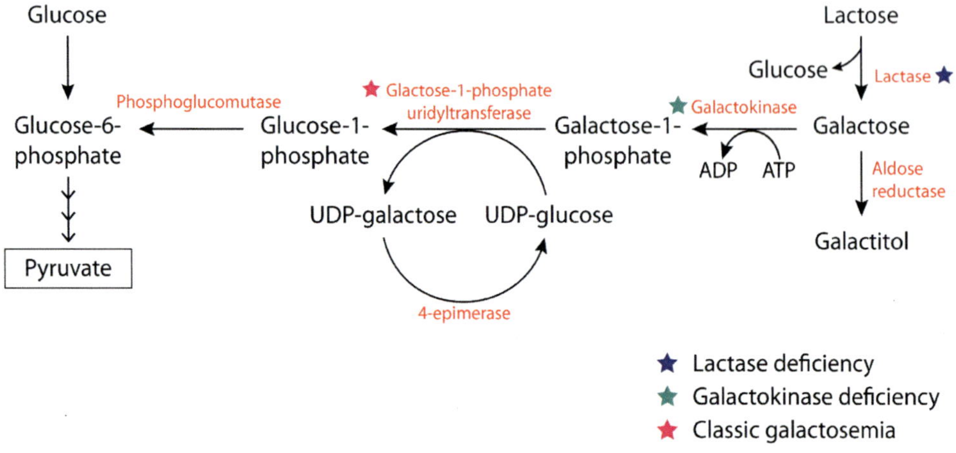

Figure 2.5.11 - Galactose

REVIEW QUESTIONS

1. A 22-year-old male was recently diagnosed with ulcerative colitis. He is treated appropriately and his symptoms resolve. However, several days later he develops flatulence, bloating, and diarrhea that seems to be worse after eating dairy products. What enzyme is most likely impaired?

   - **The patient developed secondary lactose intolerance (flatulence, bloating, and diarrhea that is worse after eating dairy products) caused by a flare up of ulcerative colitis.**
   - **Lactase is most likely impaired**

2. A 4-day-old boy is brought to the ED for vomiting. His mother states that he was born at term without any complications. Since his birth she has been exclusively breast feeding him. However, she noticed that he has become increasingly irritable and has vomited 10 times in the past 36 hours. Labs reveal hypoglycemia as well as ALT and AST elevations. A defect in carbohydrate metabolism is suspected. This patient's condition puts him at an increased risk of developing an infection by an organism that ferments what type of carbohydrate?

   - **Exclusive breast feeding resulting in hypoglycemia and liver damage (AST and ALT elevations) → classic galactosemia**
   - **This condition results in an increased risk of developing E. coli neonatal sepsis**
   - **E. coli is a gram negative rod that ferments lactose**

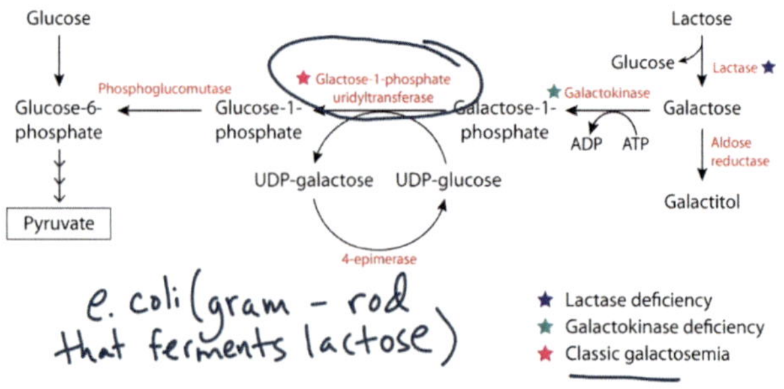

Section X - Hexose Monophosphate Pathway

I. Overview (Figure 2.5.12)

A. The HMP shunt is responsible for the synthesis of NADPH and ribose-5-phosphate (nucleotide synthesis).

B. NADPH is necessary for reductive synthetic reactions (cholesterol, steroids, and fat anabolism), protecting cells from oxidative stress, and assisting phagocytic cells (respiratory burst).

C. This pathway occurs exclusively in the cytosol.

D. Thiamine is an important cofactor for transketolase

1. ↓ thiamine → ↓ activity of HMP shunt via inhibition of transketolase

II. Fat synthesis

A. NADPH is required for the conversion of malonyl-CoA → fatty acids

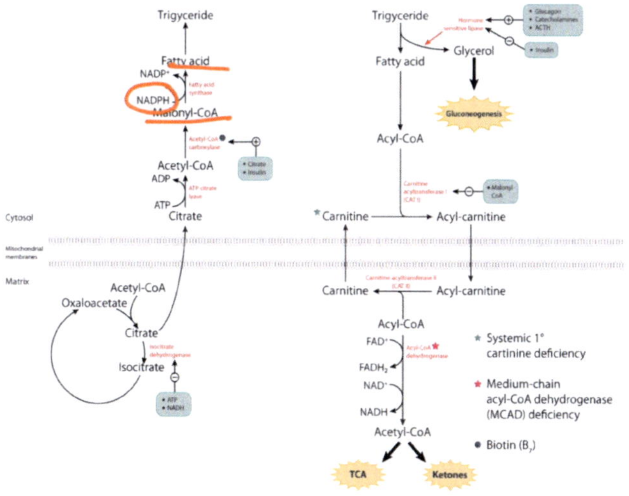

III. Glutathione

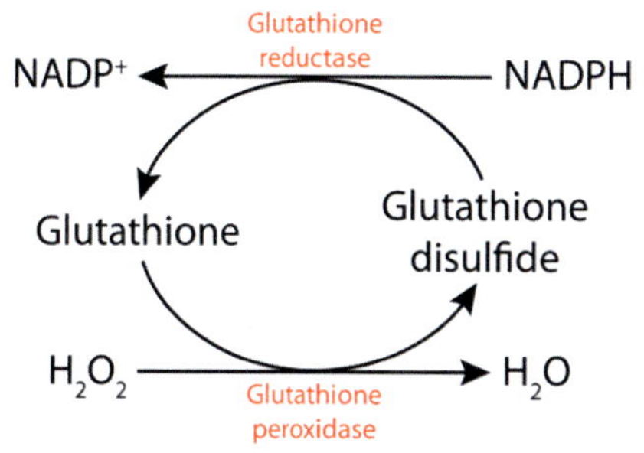

A. Protects RBCs from oxidative damage (eg, fava beans, sulfa drugs, infections) by converting H_2O_2 → H_2O

B. NADPH is necessary for the regeneration of glutathione

C. In patients with G6PD deficiency → ↓ NADPH → ↓ glutathione → ↑ oxidative damage → hemolysis

IV. Respiratory burst

A. NADPH is required for the conversion of O_2 → O_2^{-}• → weaker immune system

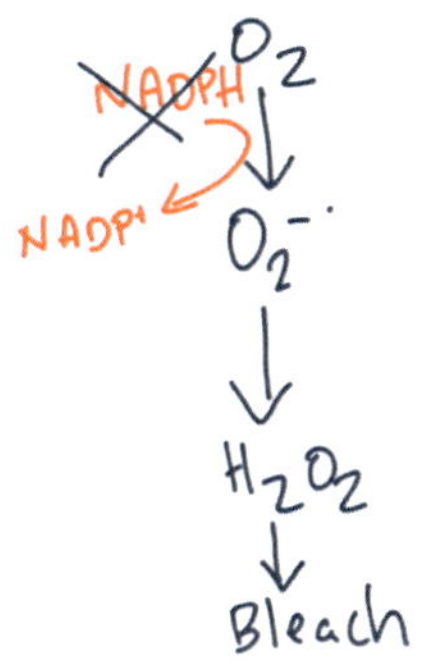

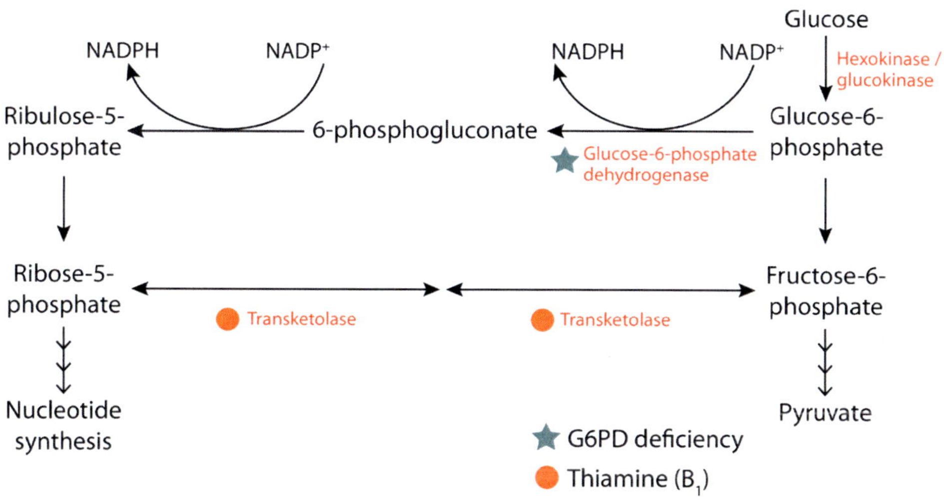

Figure 2.5.12 - HMP Shunt

REVIEW QUESTIONS

1. A 24-year-old male develops jaundice due to hemolytic anemia after digesting fava beans. A blood sample is drawn which reveals the presence of bite cells. What mechanism explains the formation of these cells?

- **Hemolytic anemia after the digestion of fava beans → G6PD deficiency**
- **G6PD deficiency → ↓ NADPH → ↓ glutathione → H_2O_2 is not able to be neutralized and reacts with hemoglobin → conglomerates of oxidized hemoglobin (Heinz bodies)**
- **As RBCs travel through the spleen the Heinz bodies are removed by splenic macrophages → development of bite cells**

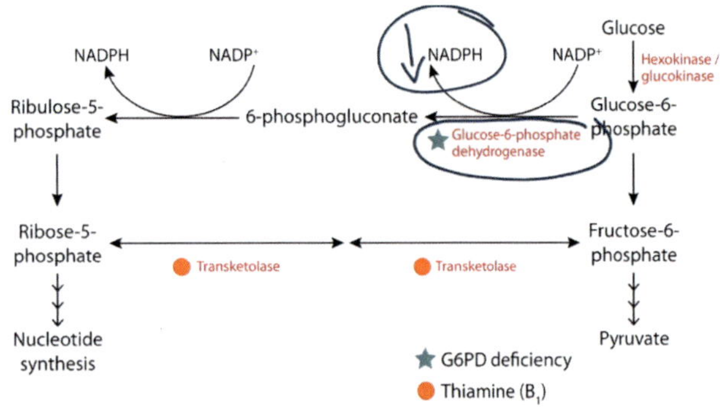

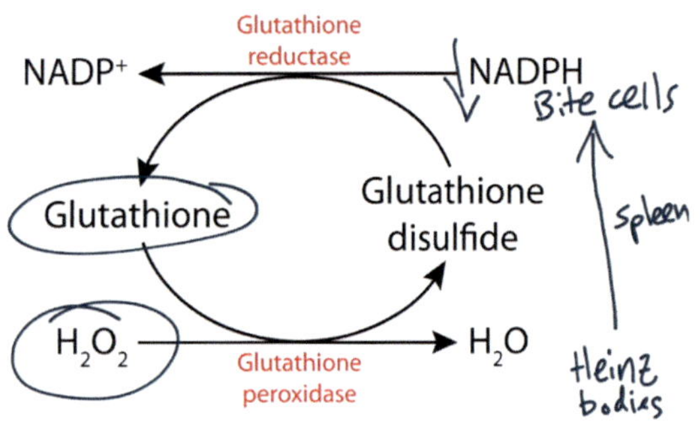

2. A patient has G6PD deficiency but is still able to synthesize nucleotides. What compensatory pathway explains this phenomenon?

- **G6PD deficiency → ↓ ribulose-5-phosphate (irreversible part of the HMP shunt)**
- **Fructose can still be converted to ribose-5-phosphate which can then be used to synthesize nucleotides due to the activity of the reversible part of the HMP shunt**

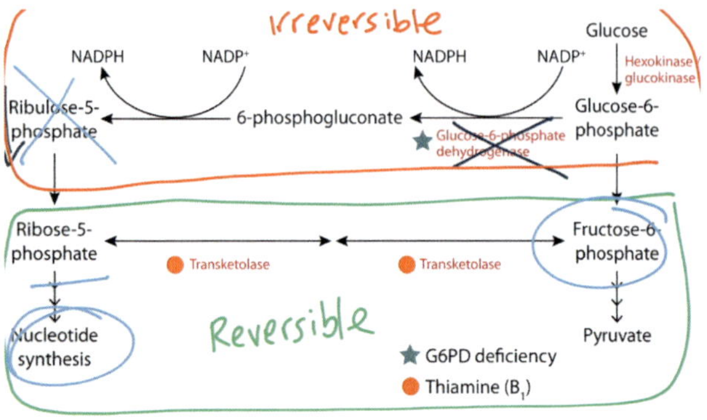

Section XI - Fatty Acid Metabolism

I. Fatty acid synthesis

A. Occurs primarily in the liver and mammary glands (primarily stored in adipocytes).

B. During high energy states ATP and NADH inhibit isocitrate dehydrogenase → ↑ citrate

C. ↑ citrate → upregulation of acetyl-CoA carboxylase (requires biotin) → ↑ fatty acid synthesis

D. Malonyl-CoA is synthesized during fatty acid synthesis and inhibits fatty acid catabolism via inhibition of carnitine acyltransferase I (CAT I).

E. NADPH (produced from the HMP shunt) is necessary for the synthesis of fatty acids.

1. HSL is activated by stress (glucagon, catecholamines, and ACTH) and inhibited by insulin.

II. Fatty acid catabolism

A. Occurs in muscle, liver, and other tissues with a mitochondrial matrix but does not occur in the brain (brain must rely on glucose and ketones) or RBCs (lack mitochondria).

B. Triglycerides are stored in adipocytes and metabolized to fatty acids and glycerol via hormone sensitive lipase (HSL).

C. Glycerol is transported to the liver to be used for gluconeogenesis.

D. Fatty acids are transported throughout the body to be used for energy in most tissues (not brain or RBCs).

E. The mitochondrial matrix is impermeable to long-chain fatty acids (LCFA). LCFAs can only enter the mitochondrial matrix through the carnitine shuttle.

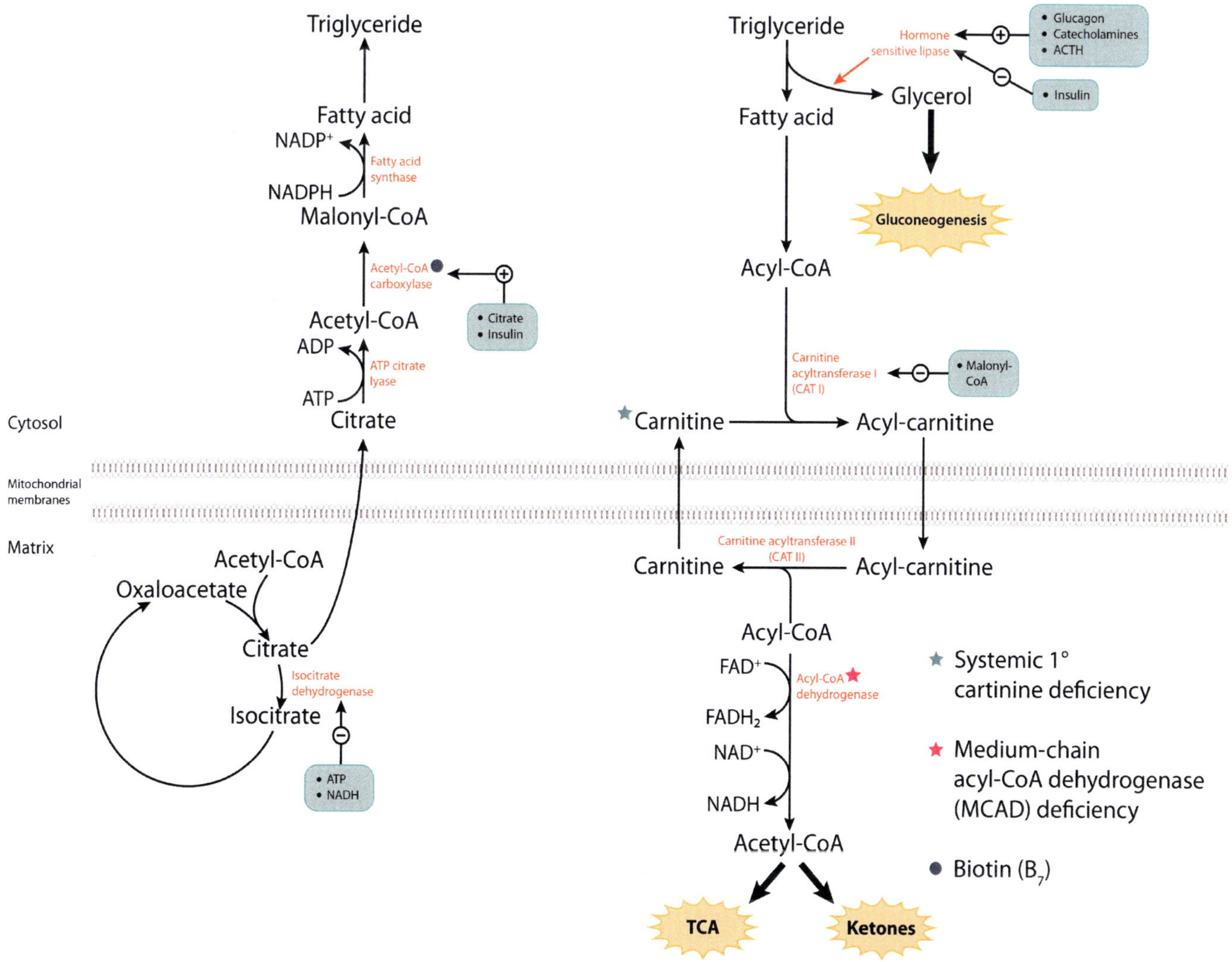

Figure 2.5.13 - Fatty acid

III. Systemic primary carnitine deficiency

A. A defect in the transporter protein that allows carnitine to be shuttled into the mitochondrial matrix.

B. The kidneys normally reabsorb carnitine and a similar defective protein in the kidneys → ↓ carnitine and acyl-carnitine

C. ↓ beta oxidation → ↓ ketones

D. ↓ acetyl-CoA → ↓ pyruvate carboxylase activity → ↓ gluconeogenesis → hypoglycemia

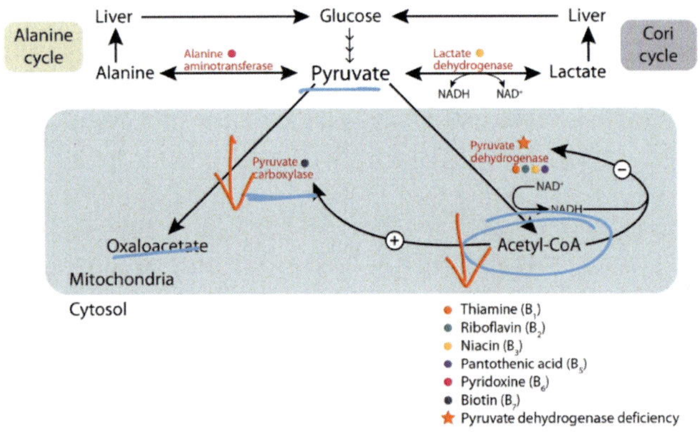

E. ↑ LCFA → liver damage → ↑ ammonia → encephalopathy

F. Treatment includes carnitine supplementation

IV. Medium-chain acyl-CoA dehydrogenase (MCAD) deficiency

A. A defective medium-chain acyl-CoA dehydrogenase

B. Similar to primary systemic carnitine deficiency (hypoketotic hypoglycemia, liver dysfunction, and encephalopathy)

C. Carnitine and acyl-carnitine levels are normal

D. LCFAs levels are normal (unless LCAD deficiency)

REVIEW QUESTIONS

1. A 26-year-old female presents with a 2-month history of constipation, depression, and kidney stones. She has also noticed white discharge from both nipples during this time and thinks she may be lactating even though she has no children. Over the past several days she has experienced several episodes of syncope. She states that several of her family members have been diagnosed with "calcium problems." An initial blood glucose measurement reveals hypoglycemia. How will the activity of carnitine acyltransferase I (CAT I) likely be altered in this patient?

- **MEN1 (pituitary, pancreatic, and parathyroid tumors)**
- **Parathyroid adenoma → hypercalcemia → constipation, depression, and kidney stones**
- **Prolactinoma → white discharge from both nipples**
- **Insulinoma → several episodes of syncope due to hypoglycemia**
- **Insulin increases the activity of acetyl-CoA carboxylase → ↑ malonyl-CoA → inhibition of carnitine acyltransferase I**

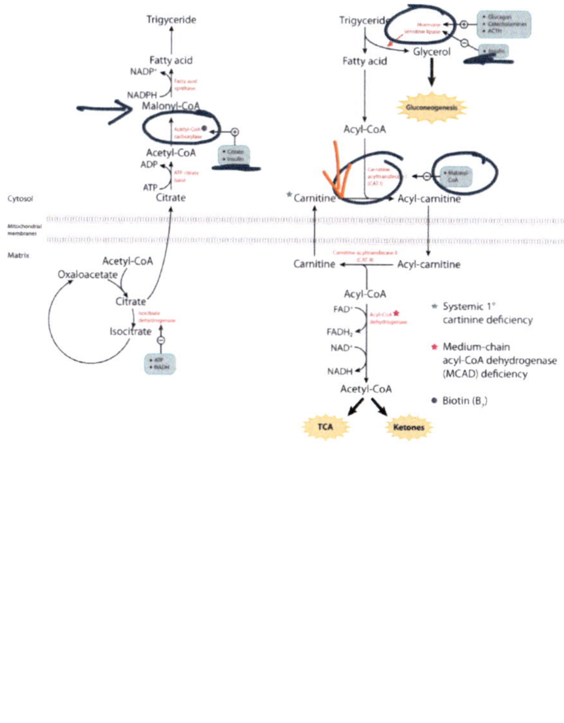

2. A previously healthy 10-year-old Jewish boy is brought to the ED by his mother who states that he developed nausea and vomiting followed by a syncopal episode after participating in a fast for Yom Kippur. Labs are significant for hypoglycemia and non-detectable levels of acetoacetate. A muscle biopsy reveals normal levels of a protein responsible for transporting long-chain fatty acids into the mitochondrial matrix. It is determined that impairment of gluconeogenesis likely resulted in hypoglycemia. Decreased activity of what enzyme involved in gluconeogenesis most likely explains these findings?

- **Hypoketotic hypoglycemia during a fast → MCAD deficiency or systemic primary carnitine deficiency**
- **"A muscle biopsy reveals normal levels of a protein responsible for transporting long-chain fatty acids into the mitochondrial matrix" is describing carnitine → patient does not have systemic primary carnitine deficiency**
- **MCAD deficiency → ↓ acetyl-CoA → ↓ pyruvate carboxylase → hypoglycemia**

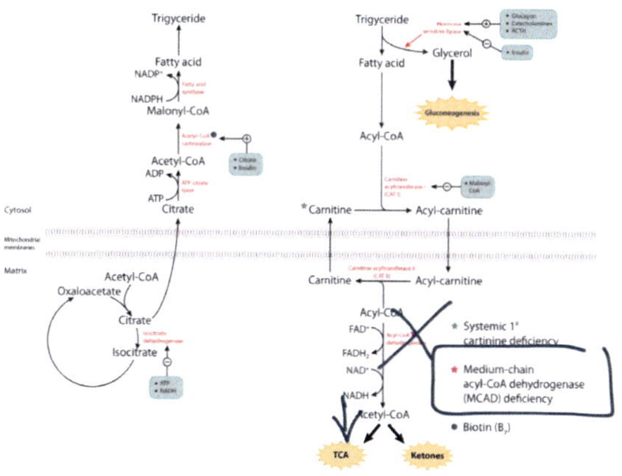

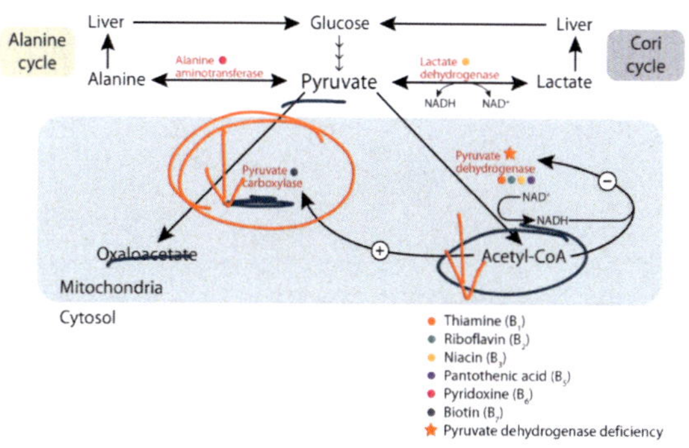

Section XII - Ketone Bodies

I. Overview

A. The brain cannot metabolize fatty acids directly. Ketone bodies can be produced from fatty acids by the liver and then utilized by the brain during times of starvation.

B. Ketone body synthesis acts as an overflow pathway for acetyl-CoA in the liver during times of excessive fatty acid catabolism.

C. RBCs and hepatocytes cannot use ketones.

D. Synthesis is upregulated during intense gluconeogenesis (fasting, carbohydrate restricted diet, intense exercise, type I diabetes, etc.).

II. Type I Diabetics

A. ↓ insulin → ↑ gluconeogenesis → depletion of oxaloacetate → TCA cycle inhibition → ↑ acetyl-CoA → ↑ ketone body synthesis

III. Ethanol

A. ↑ NADH → oxaloacetate shunted to malate → ↑ acetyl-CoA → ↑ ketone body synthesis

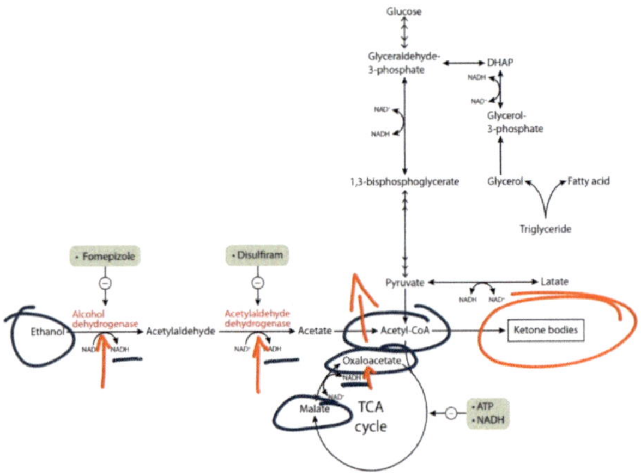

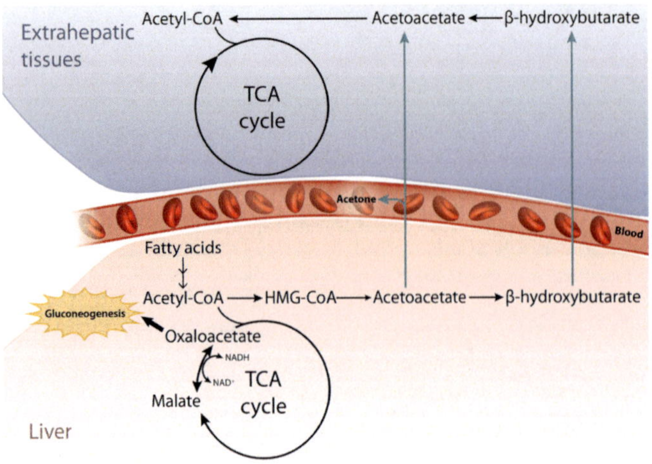

Figure 2.5.14 - Ketones

REVIEW QUESTIONS

1. What two cell types are unable to utilize ketone bodies as an energy source?

   - **RBCs (lack mitochondria) and hepatocytes (produces ketones for other tissues)**

2. A 21-year-old male presents to the ED with sudden onset abdominal pain, nausea, and vomiting. He states that he developed an upper respiratory infection several weeks ago which has since resolved. He is otherwise healthy with no significant past medical history. His exam is significant for tachypnea, diffuse abdominal pain, and a fruity breath odor. Labs reveal a blood glucose level of 587 mg/dL. Depletion of what intermediate in the TCA cycle is likely responsible for the fruity breath odor detected on physical examination?

   - **Abdominal pain, tachypnea, fruity breath odor, and a blood glucose level of 587 mg/dL → diabetic ketoacidosis**
   - **↓ insulin → ↑ gluconeogenesis → depletion of oxaloacetate → TCA cycle inhibition → ↑ acetyl-CoA → ↑ ketone body synthesis**

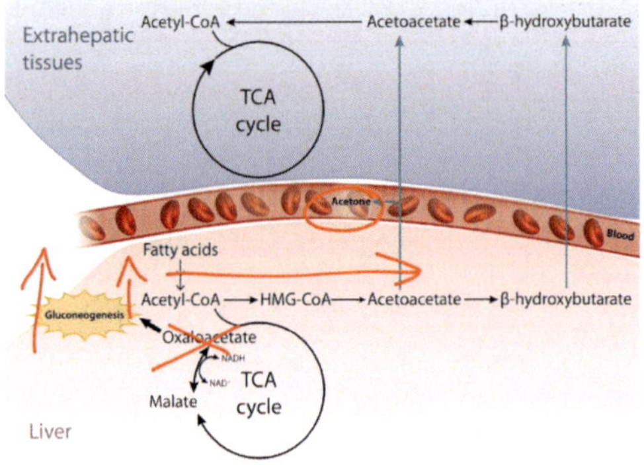

Section XIII - Ethanol Metabolism

I. Ethanol is converted into acetyl-CoA and results in the production of NADH.

II. Many of the symptoms seen in alcoholism can be explained by elevated levels of NADH.

   A. ↑ NADH → ↓ oxaloacetate → ↓ gluconeogenesis → hypoglycemia

   B. ↑ NADH/ATP → inhibition of TCA cycle → ↑ acetyl-CoA → ↑ ketone body synthesis

   C. ↑ NADH/ATP → inhibition of TCA cycle → ↑ acetyl-CoA → ↑ pyruvate → ↑ lactate → lactic acidosis

   D. ↑ NADH → ↑ glycerol-3-phosphate → ↑ triglycerides → hepatosteatosis

III. Enzymes of ethanol metabolism

   A. Alcohol dehydrogenase

      1. Inhibited by fomepizole (used to treat methanol and ethylene glycol intoxication).

   B. Acetaldehyde dehydrogenase

      1. Inhibited by disulfiram (can be used to deter alcoholics from consuming alcohol).

IV. Alcoholism causes malabsorption and malnutrition resulting in thiamine deficiency. Thiamine is a necessary cofactor for several enzymes.

   A. Pyruvate dehydrogenase

   B. α-ketoglutarate dehydrogenase

   C. Transketolase

   D. Branched-chain ketoacid dehydrogenase

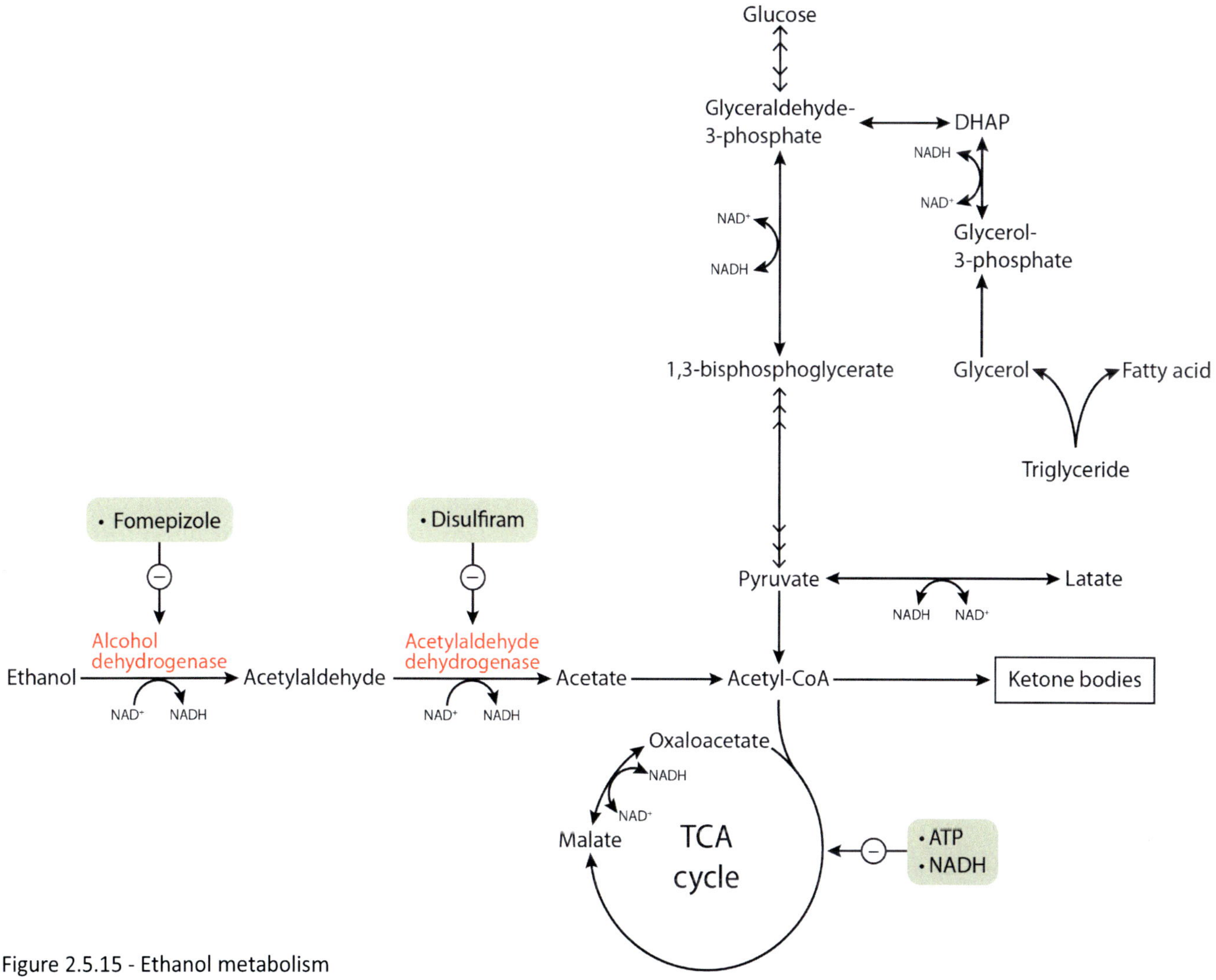

Figure 2.5.15 - Ethanol metabolism

REVIEW QUESTIONS

1. A 65-year-old male presents to clinic for a routine evaluation. Physical exam is significant for mild hepatomegaly. Labs reveal an AST of 230 and an ALT of 115. This patient's physical exam and lab findings are most likely due to impaired gluconeogenesis resulting in an accumulation of what metabolite in hepatocytes?

- **An AST:ALT ratio 2:1 is suggestive of alcoholic-related liver damage**
- **Alcoholism → ↑ NADH → ↑ glycerol-3-phosphate → ↑ triglycerides → hepatosteatosis**

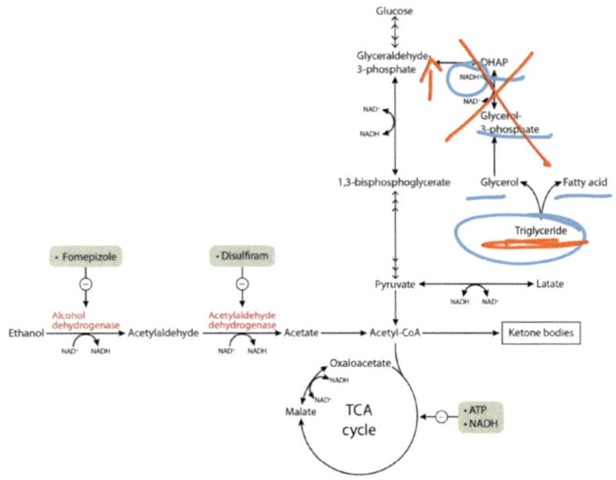

2. A 41-year-old homeless male is brought to the ED after being found unconscious in the street. The individual who brought him to the hospital stated that he smelled of alcohol. After proper resuscitation it is determined that he has a vitamin deficiency resulting in memory problems. What enzyme involved in the synthesis of DNA is likely impaired as a result of this patient's vitamin deficiency?

- **Chronic alcohol use → memory problems**
- **Chronic alcohol use can cause thiamine deficiency → necessary cofactor for transketolase (necessary for nucleotide synthesis / DNA synthesis)**

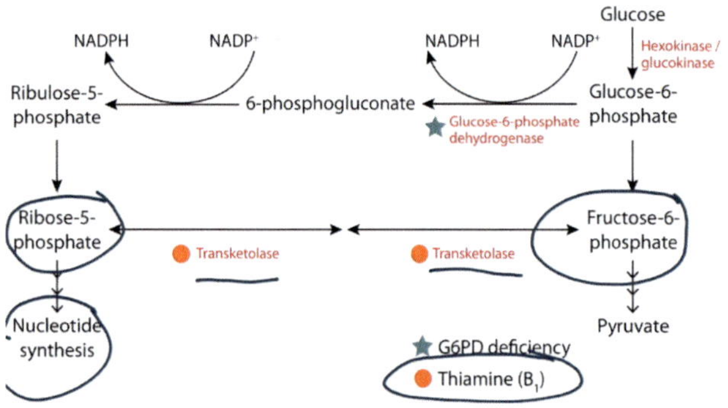

Section XIV - Lipid Transport

I. Cholesterol synthesis occurs exclusively in the liver.

   A. Acetyl-CoA → cholesterol

   B. Rate limiting step is HMG-CoA reductase

II. Because fat is not soluble in water, it must be transported in the blood by lipoproteins (lipid-protein complexes).

   A. Chylomicrons

      1. Produced by enterocytes and transport fatty acids and cholesterol to the tissues.

      2. B-48: necessary for chylomicron secretion from enterocytes

         a) Mnemonic: He 8 cholesterol

      3. ApoC-II: cofactor for lipoprotein lipase

         a) Mnemonic: C = cofactor

   B. Very low-density lipoprotein (VLDL)

      1. Produced by the liver and transports fatty acids and cholesterol to the tissues.

      2. As VLDL loses fatty acids → IDL

      3. ApoE: facilitates binding of chylomicrons, VLDL, intermediate-density lipoprotein (IDL), and high-density lipoprotein (HDL) to the hepatic remnant receptors

         a) Mnemonic: E = everything; rEmnant

      4. ApoB-100: necessary for hepatic secretion of VLDL and facilitates binding of LDL to hepatic low-density lipoprotein (LDL) receptors

      5. ApoC-II: cofactor for lipoprotein lipase

      6. ApoE: facilitates binding of chylomicrons, VLDL, IDL, and HDL to the hepatic remnant receptors

   C. LDL

      1. Delivers cholesterol to periphery

      2. Only contains ApoB-100

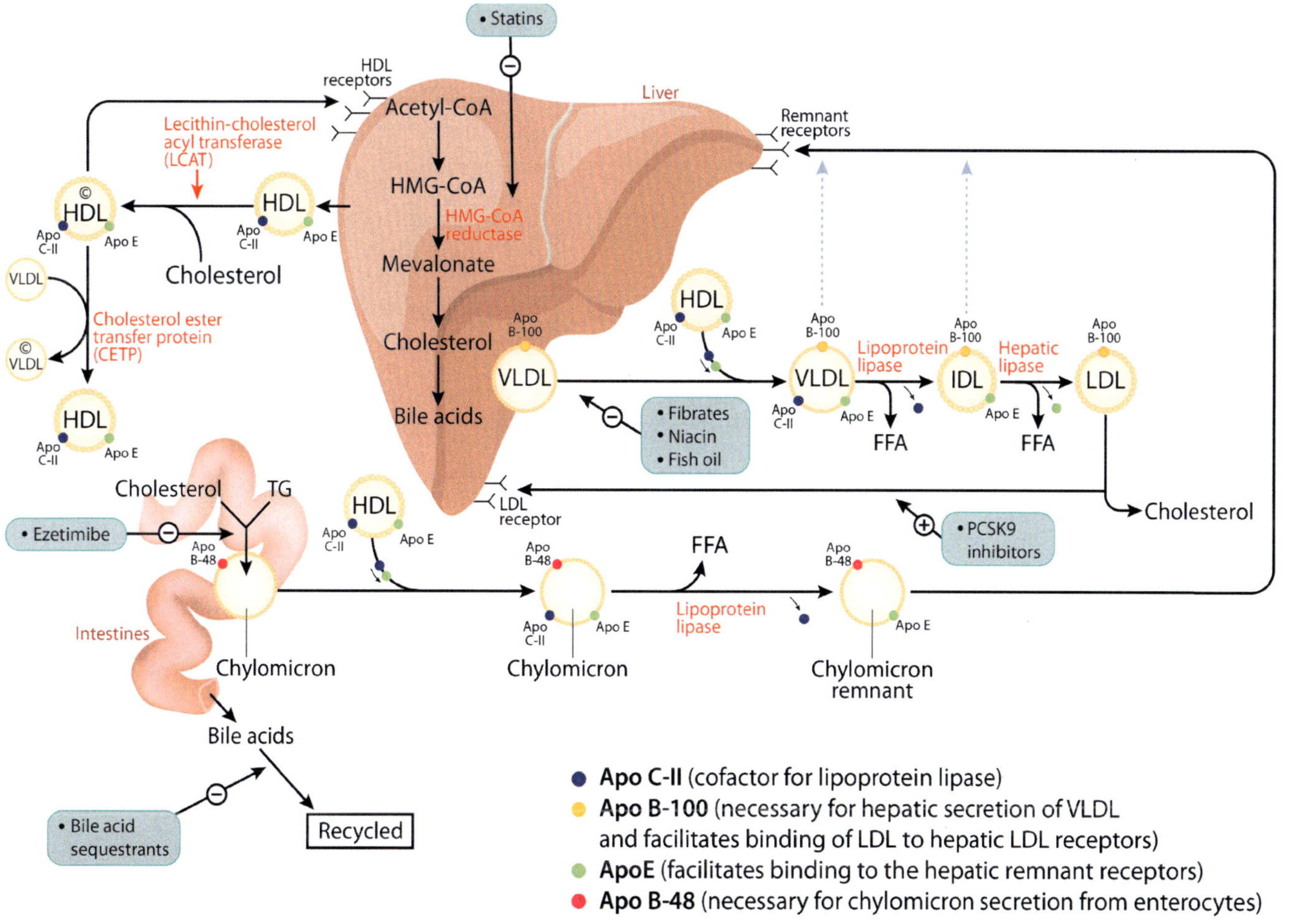

Figure 2.5.16 - Lipid transport

D. HDL removes cholesterol from the periphery and delivers it to the liver.

1. Lecithin-cholesterol acyl transferase (LCAT) converts cholesterol from the periphery into esterified cholesterol → densely packed into HDL core.
2. Cholesterol ester transfer protein (CETP) transfers cholesterol esters to other lipoproteins (i.e. VLDL, LDL, etc.).
3. HDL contains ApoE which facilitates hepatic uptake of HDL.
4. Also contains ApoC-II and ApoA-I.

III. Measuring cholesterol

A. Lipid panel: LDL, HDL, and VLDL

B. VLDL transports a high concentration of triglycerides

C. VLDL used as a surrogate for triglycerides

IV. Familial dyslipidemias (Figure 2.5.17)

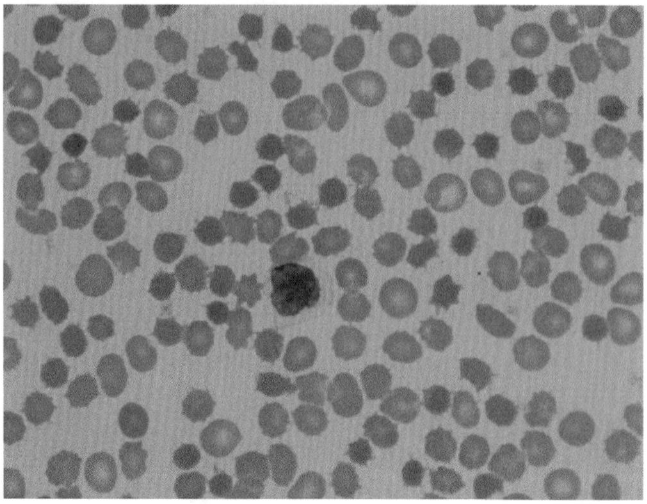

Figure 2.5.17 - Spur cell

Dyslipidemia	Protein defect(s)	Labs	Findings
Abetalipoproteinemia	• Inability to synthesize ApoB-100 (absence → inability to secrete VLDL from liver) and ApoB-48 (necessary for chylomicron secretion from enterocytes)	• ↓ Chylomicrons • ↓ VLDL • ↓ IDL • ↓ LDL	Fat soluble vitamin deficiency Acanthocytosis
Familial hyperchylomicronemia (type I)	• Apo C-II (a cofactor for LPL) • LPL	• ↑ Triglycerides (chylomicrons and VLDL)	Xanthomas Pancreatitis
Familial hypercholesterolemia (type II)	• ApoB-100 defect (allows VLDL and associated remnants to bind to the LDL receptor on hepatocytes) • LDL receptor	• ↑ LDL	Xanthomas Coronary disease
Familial dysbetalipoproteinemia (type III)	• ApoE3 & ApoE4 (allows chylomicrons, VLDL, and IDL to bind to hepatic lipoprotein receptors)	• ↑ Triglycerides (chylomicrons, VLDL, and IDL)	Xanthomas Coronary disease
Familial hypertriglyceridemia (type IV)	• Overproduction of VLDL	• ↑ Triglycerides (VLDL)	Xanthomas (rare) Pancreatitis Coronary disease

Table 2.5.2 - Familial dyslipidemias

REVIEW QUESTIONS

1. A 16-year-old female is brought to the physician by her father due to worsening vision over the past two weeks. He states that she has a history of mild cognitive impairment and diarrhea. Fundoscopy reveals bilateral retinitis pigmentosa. Laboratory findings are significant for low levels of total serum cholesterol. What apolipoproteins are most likely deficient in this patient?

   - **Worsening vision, bilateral retinitis pigmentosa, and low levels of total serum cholesterol → abetalipoproteinemia**
   - **Characterized by a deficiency of ApoB-48 and ApoB-100 → ↓ chylomicrons, VLDL, IDL, and LDL**
   - **Vision changes caused by a deficiency of vitamin A**
   - **Neurological changes caused by a deficiency of vitamin E**
   - **Diarrhea caused by fat accumulation in the bowel**

2. A 24-year-old male presents for a routine visit. On exam he is noted to have yellow nodules on the flexor tendons of his hands and feet. His total serum cholesterol and LDL are elevated. His triglyceride levels are normal. What apolipoprotein is most likely defective in this patient?

   - **Xanthomas (yellow nodules) are suggestive of a dyslipidemia**
   - **Elevated LDL and normal triglyceride levels → type II dyslipidemia**
   - **Caused by a defect in ApoB-100 or the LDL receptor**

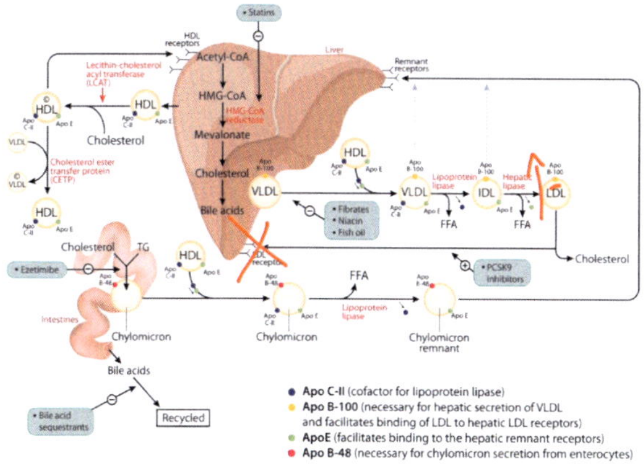

3. A 65-year-old male presents to the ED with sudden onset left-sided weakness. He has facial droop and slurred speech. He is started on several medications including atorvastatin. How will this drug likely alter the number of LDL receptors on hepatocytes?

   - **Statins (atorvastatin) inhibit HMG-CoA reductase → ↓ hepatic cholesterol concentration → ↑ LDL receptor expression in attempt to restore hepatic cholesterol levels back to normal**

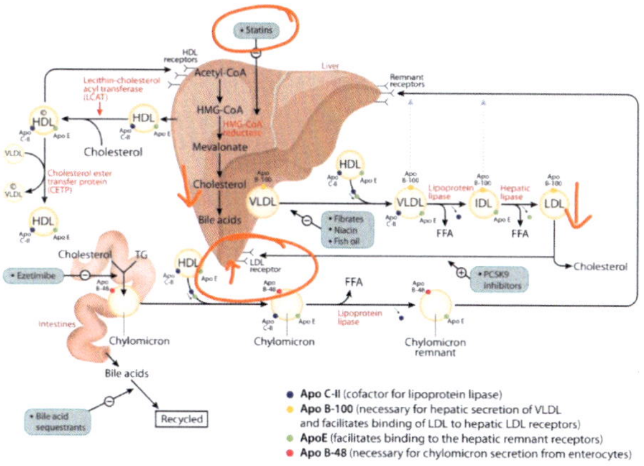

Section XV - Homocysteine Metabolism

I. Homocystinuria (Figure 2.5.18)

A. Most commonly due to a deficiency of cystathionine synthase

B. ↑ homocysteine in urine

C. Cysteine becomes an essential amino acid

D. Symptoms include intellectual disability, hypercoagulability, ectopia lentis (lens displacement), and a marfanoid habitus.

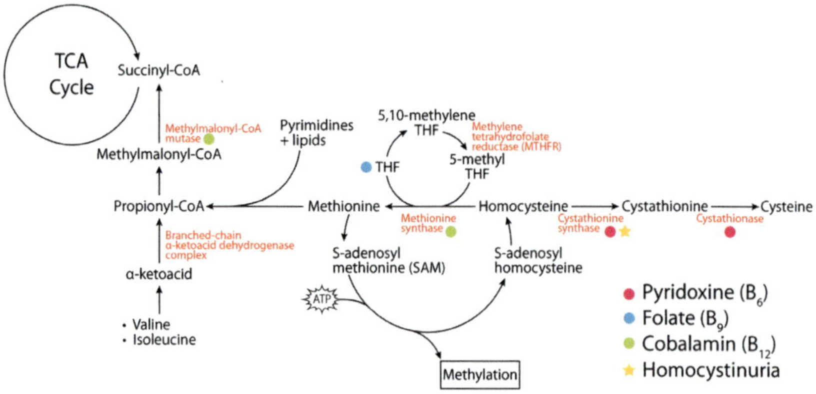

Figure 2.5.18 - Homocysteine metabolism

II. Vitamin B_{12} (cobalamin)

A. Necessary for the conversion of homocysteine → methionine and methylmalonyl-CoA → succinyl-CoA

B. Deficiency results in ↑ methylmalonic acid (MMA) and homocysteine

III. Vitamin B_9 (folate)

A. Necessary for the conversion of homocysteine → methionine

B. Deficiency results in ↑ homocysteine and normal levels of MMA

REVIEW QUESTIONS

1. A 4-year-old boy is brought to the physician by his mother due to swelling in his leg. The mother states that his symptoms developed yesterday. Since then the boy has complained of difficulty walking. On exam he is noted to be intellectually delayed. He is in the 99th percentile for height and his limbs are especially elongated. Labs reveal elevated cystathionine and homocysteine. A deficiency of what enzyme is most likely responsible for this patient's condition?

   - **Marfanoid habitus (elongated limbs), intellectual disability, DVTs, and elevated cystathionine and homocysteine → homocystinuria**
   - **Elevated cystathionine and homocysteine → deficiency of methionine synthase**

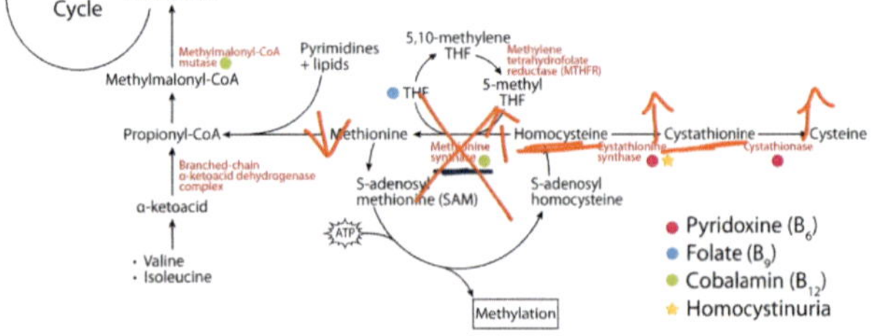

2. A homeless male presents to the ED with a constellation of symptoms and the physician on call is concerned about a vitamin deficiency. Labs are ordered and reveal elevated levels of homocysteine and normal levels of methylmalonic acid. Supplementation with what vitamin would likely improve this patient's condition?

   - **↑ homocysteine and normal levels of methylmalonic acid → folate deficiency (supplementation with folate would improve this patient's condition)**

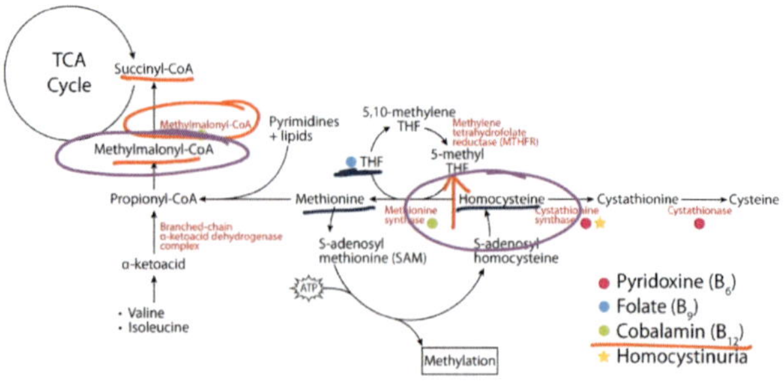

Section XVI - Purines & Pyrimidines

I. Overview

A. Nitrogenous bases (purines and pyrimidines) are used to synthesize DNA and RNA.

B. Purines: adenine and guanine

C. Pyrimidines: cytosine, thymine, and uracil

II. Purine synthesis

A. Ribose-5-phosphate → adenine and guanine

III. Pyrimidine synthesis

A. Ribose-5-phosphate → cytosine, thymine, and uracil

B. Orotic aciduria

1. Deficiency of UMP synthase
2. Megaloblastic anemia
3. No hyperammonemia
4. Treatment is uridine supplementation

C. The synthesis of dTMP requires folate.

IV. Purine salvage pathway

A. Allows purines to be recycled in order to conserve energy.

B. Free bases are converted back into GMP, IMP, and AMP for use in DNA and RNA synthesis.

C. Adenosine deaminase deficiency results in the accumulation of adenosine metabolites in T-lymphocytes → severe combined immunodeficiency disease (SCID)

D. The salvage pathway requires the enzyme hypoxanthine gaunine phosphoribosyltransferase (HGPRT).

E. Elimination of purines in the form of uric acid is implicated in the pathogenesis of gout.

F. Lesch-Nyhan syndrome

1. Deficiency of HGPRT enzyme
2. ↑ uric acid production → gout
3. Self-mutilation
4. Intellectual disability

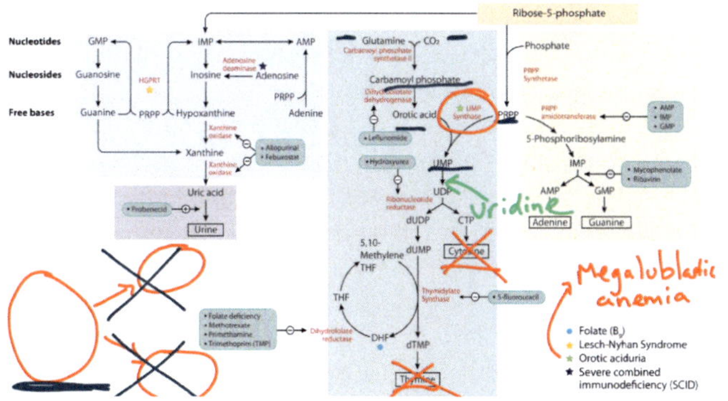

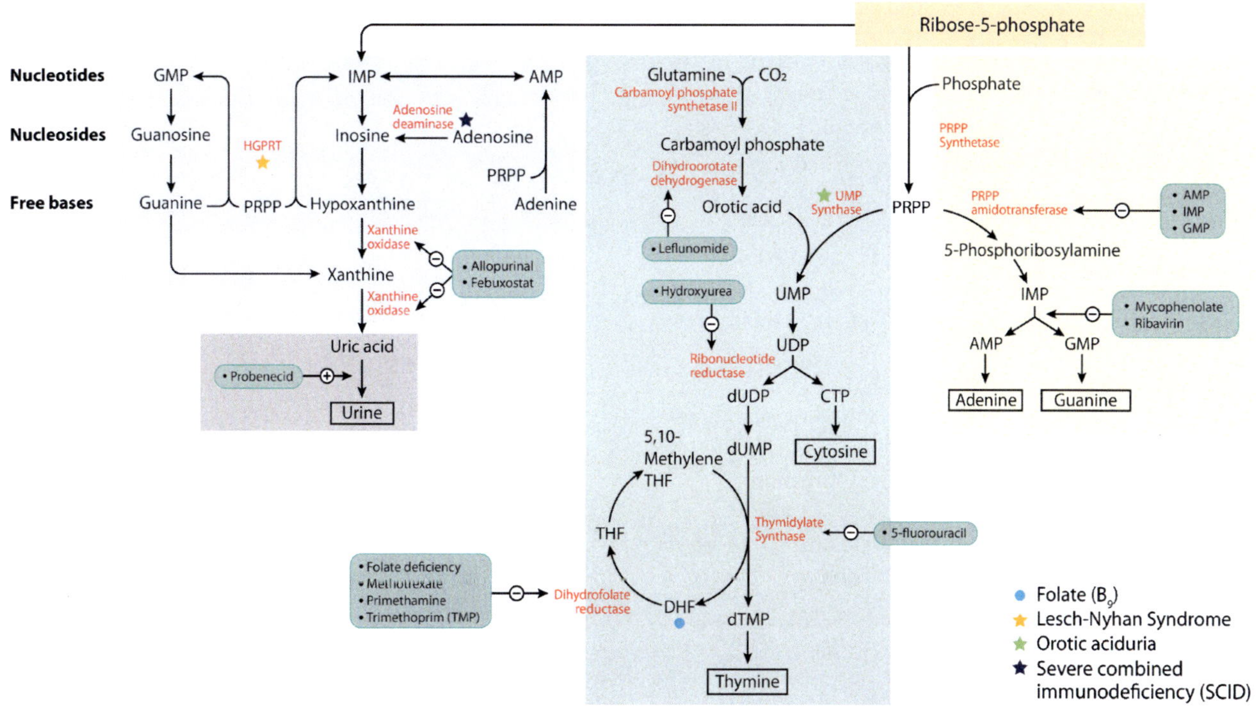

Figure 2.5.19 - Nucleotides

REVIEW QUESTIONS

1. A 7-year-old boy is brought to the physician by his mother who states that he has had two months of worsening fatigue. When asked about the boy's diet his mother states that the family is vegan. However, she is adamant that they supplement his diet with all of the vitamins he needs for proper development including cobalamin and folate. A CBC reveals anemia with an MCV of 100. This patient's anemia is likely a result of a deficiency of what enzyme?

- **Macrocytic anemia (MCV >100) in conjunction with cobalamin and folate supplementation makes B_{12} and folate deficiencies less likely**
- **Orotic aciduria can cause a macrocytic anemia (thymine and cytosine are not synthesized which are necessary for DNA synthesis)**
- **Caused by a deficiency of UMP synthase**

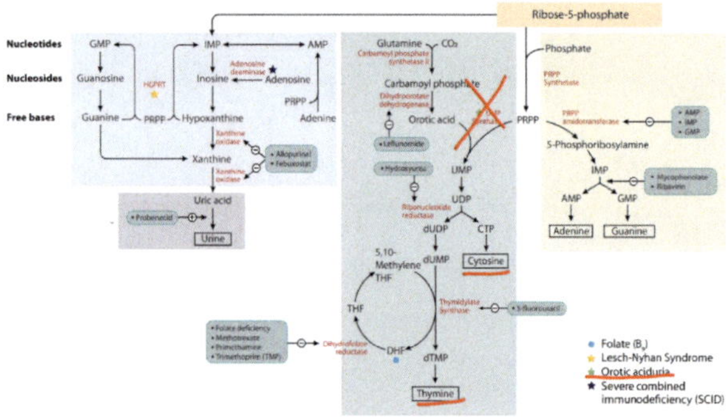

2. A 42-year-old female with a past medical history significant for multiple psychiatric hospital admissions presents with recent onset fatigue. She is accompanied by her brother who states that her eating habits have been quite eccentric. A CBC reveals anemia with an MCV of 118. Homocysteine levels are elevated but methylmalonic acid levels are normal. What two supplements are likely to improve this patient's anemia?

- **Macrocytic anemia, eccentric eating habits, elevated homocysteine levels, and normal methylmalonic acid (MMA) levels → folate deficiency**
- **B_{12} deficiency results in ↑ MMA**
- **Folate deficiency results in ↑ homocysteine and normal MMA**
- **A folate deficiency results in ↓ thymine synthesis**
- **Supplementation with thymine and folate would likely improve this patient's anemia**

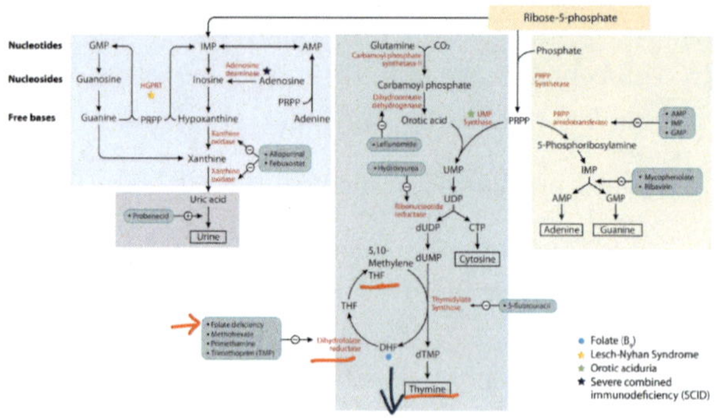

3. A 4-year-old boy presents with painful swollen wrists. His mother states that he has had multiple episodes similar to this. Upon further discussion, the physician discovers that the boy is severely intellectually delayed and has had multiple episodes of self-mutilation. An enzyme deficiency is suspected and confirmed with appropriate laboratory tests. How will the activity of transketolase likely be altered in this patient?

- **Gout, intellectual disability, and self-mutilation → Lesch-Nyhan syndrome**
- **Deficiency of HGPRT → ↓ recycling of purines → ↑ synthesis of de novo purines**
- **Transketolase generates ribose-5-phosphate (precursor to de novo synthesis pathway) so this enzyme will most likely be upregulated**

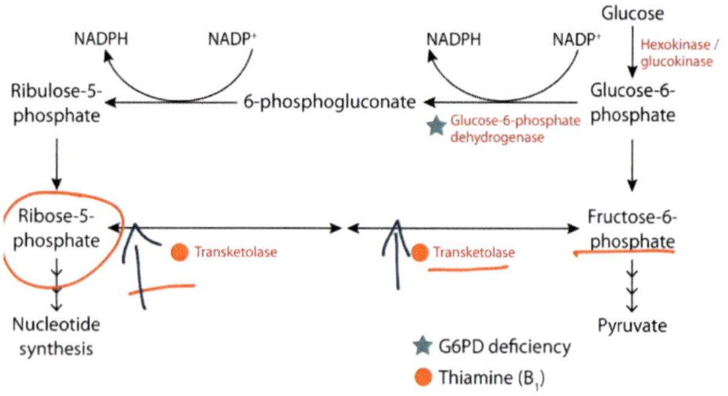

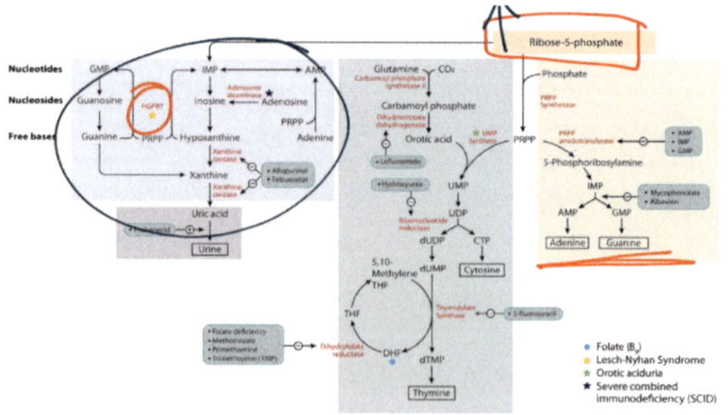

Section XVII - Ammonia

I. Overview

A. The catabolism of proteins results in NH3 production.

B. Free NH3 is a toxic substance. It must be transported to the liver where it can be converted into urea via the urea cycle and then removed from the body in the form of urine.

II. Alanine cycle

A. A coordinated series of reactions that occurs between the muscle and the liver and allows amino acids to be used as energy.

III. Urea cycle (Figure 2.5.20)

A. One of the major pathways for the disposal of nitrogen waste (i.e. catabolism of amino acids).

B. Most defects in the pathway → ↑ ammonia → neurotoxicity.

C. Carbamoyl phosphate synthetase I is the rate-limiting step.

D. Ornithine transcarbamylase deficiency is caused by a deficiency of ornithine transcarbamylase.

1. ↓ urea cycle activity → symptoms of hyperammonemia

2. ↑ orotic acid (funneled to pyrimidine pathway)

IV. Hyperammonemia (Figure 2.5.21)

A. Caused by liver disease or urea cycle disorders.

B. Neurological symptoms develop (slurred speech, asterixis, tremors, somnolence, and encephalopathy).

1. ↑ NH_3 → ↑ glutamine in astrocytes → osmotic impairment of glutamine release → ↓ glutamine in neurons → ↓ glutamate in neurons → encephalopathy

C. Treatment includes lactulose and rifaximin.

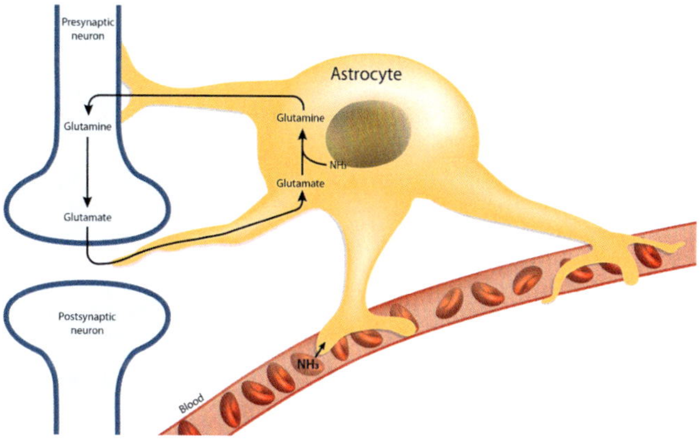

Figure 2.5.21 - Astrocytes

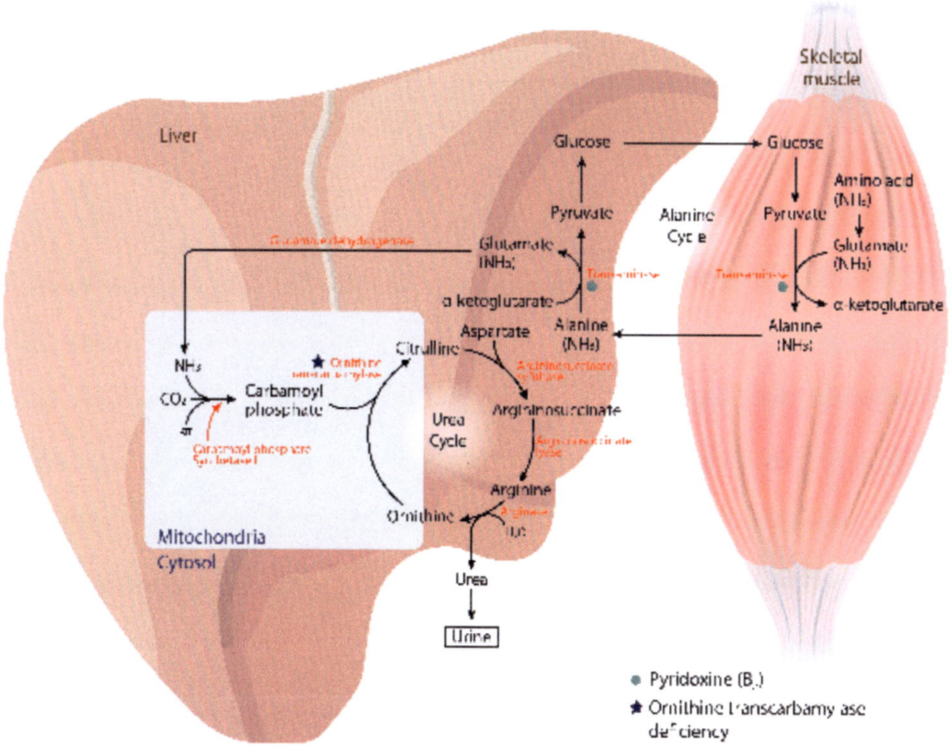

Figure 2.5.20 - Urea cycle

REVIEW QUESTIONS

1. A 51-year-old homeless male presents to the ED with slurred speech. On exam he has asterixis and is encephalopathic. Alcohol-related liver damage is suspected. Labs are significant for transaminitis including an ALT of 200 U/L (normal: 8-20). This enzyme is responsible for transferring the amino group from alanine to what compound?

    - **ALT is a transaminase enzyme that converts alanine → pyruvate**
    - **α-ketoglutarate receives the amino group from alanine**

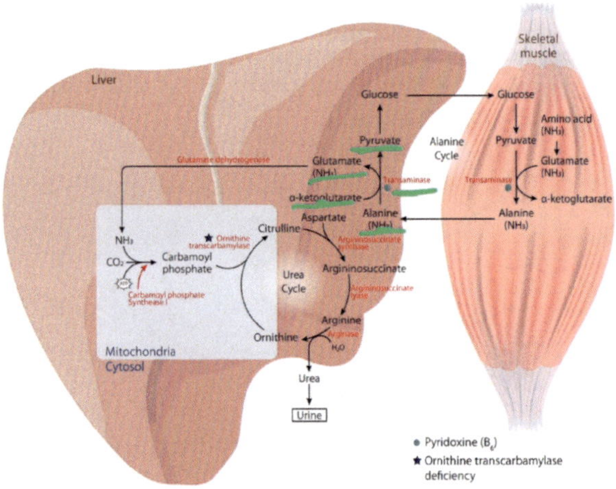

2. A 1-year-old boy is brought to the physician due to worsening episodes of somnolence. Labs are significant for hyperammonemia and increased orotic acid in the urine. A deficiency of an enzyme responsible for synthesizing citrulline is suspected. How would the activity of UMP synthase likely be altered in this patient?

    - **Hyperammonemia and ↑ orotic acid → urea cycle disorder**
    - **The deficient enzyme normally synthesizes citrulline → ornithine transcarbamylase is deficient → ↑ carbamoyl phosphate**
    - **Carbamoyl phosphate is also used during the synthesis of pyrimidines and gets converted to orotic acid (hence the elevated orotic acid) → ↑ activity of UMP synthase**

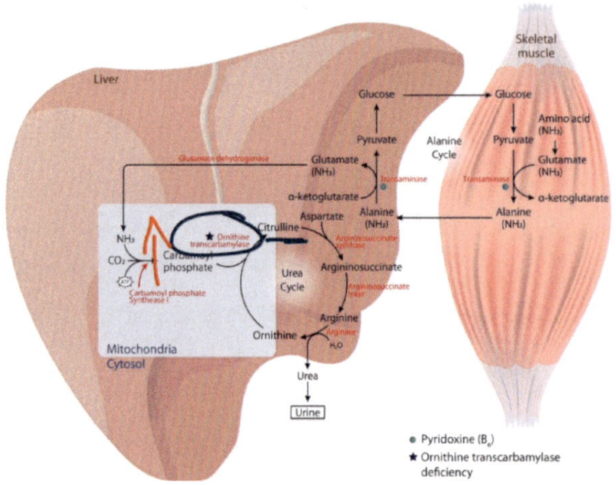

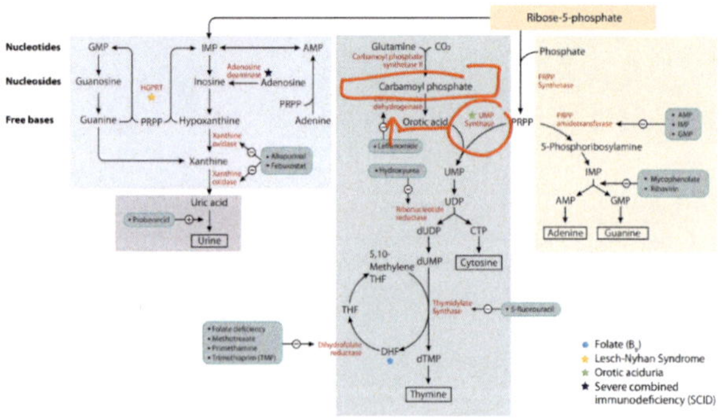

Section XVIII - Amino Acids

I. Maple syrup urine disease (Figure 2.5.22)

A. An autosomal recessive disorder resulting in defective metabolism of branched-chain amino acids (isoleucine, leucine, and valine).

B. Deficiency of branched-chain α-ketoacid dehydrogenase complex (BCKDC) → ↑ α-ketoacids.

1. BCKDC requires 5 cofactors including thiamine (vitamin B_1), lipoic acid, coenzyme A (vitamin B_5), FAD (vitamin B_2), and NAD (vitamin B_3).

2. Mnemonic: "TLC for Nancy."

C. Isoleucine metabolites in the urine → maple syrup / burnt sugar smell in the urine.

D. Results in neurological symptoms (intellectual disability, seizures, irritability).

II. Phenylketonuria (Figure 2.5.23)

A. Caused by a deficiency of phenylalanine hydroxylase or dihydrobiopterin reductase.

B. Results in a downstream deficiency of neurotransmitters.

C. Symptoms include seizures, intellectual disability, and a "musty" odor.

D. Treatment varies depending on specific deficiency.

III. Catecholamine synthesis

A. Phenylalanine is necessary for the synthesis of DOPA.

B. DOPA is converted to dopamine via DOPA decarboxylase.

C. Carbidopa inhibits DOPA decarboxylase and can be used to treat Parkinson's disease.

D. The conversion of norepinephrine to epinephrine is catalyzed by the enzyme phenylethanolamine-N-methyltransferase (PNMT).

E. PMNT is upregulated by cortisol.

IV. Albinism

A. Due to a deficiency of tyrosinase

B. ↓ melanin synthesis

C. Normal melanocyte number

D. ↑ risk of skin cancer

V. Alkaptonuria

A. Deficiency of homogentisic acid dioxygenase

B. ↑ homogentisic acid → pigmented deposition occurs in connective tissue.

C. Deposition occurs in joints → arthritis

D. Homogentisic acid in urine is oxidized by air → black urine

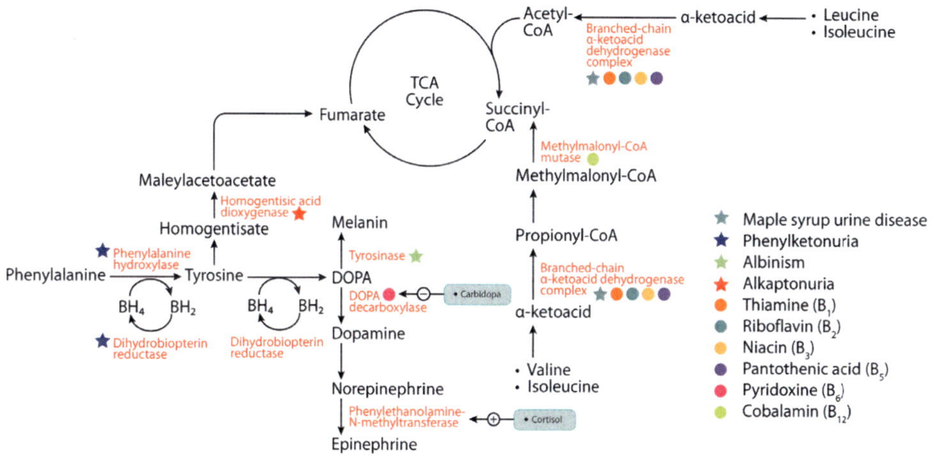

Figure 2.5.22 - Amino acids

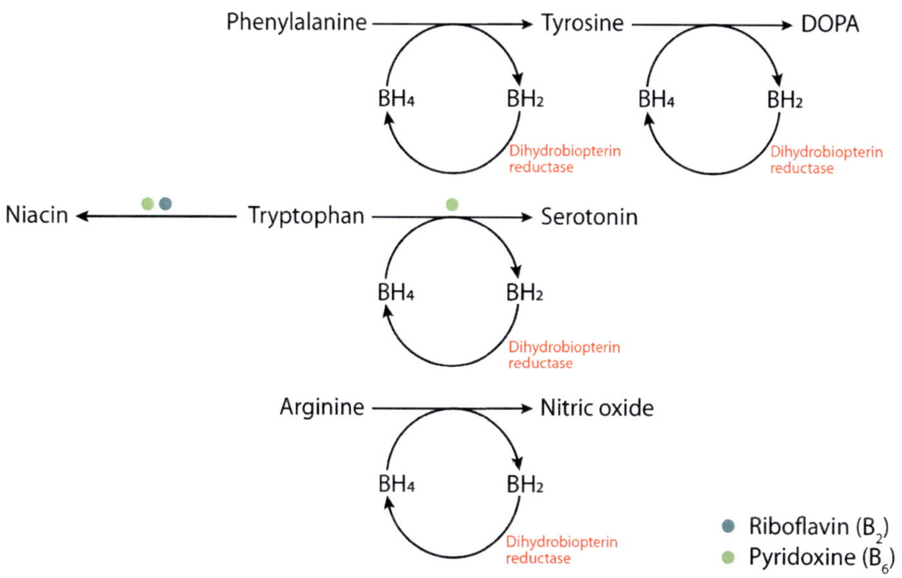

Figure 2.5.23 - BH_4

REVIEW QUESTIONS

1. An 8-month-old boy is brought to the physician by his mother for seizures. She states that she hasn't recognized any prior seizure activity until recently, but notes that he has been very irritable since birth compared to her other children. A sweet smell is noted while changing the boy's diaper during a brief genital exam. An enzyme deficiency is suspected as the cause of this patient's symptoms. Based on your understanding of the most likely deficient enzyme, what supplements may be helpful in improving this patient's condition?

- **Neurological deficits and a sweet smell in the urine → maple syrup urine disease (MSUD)**
- **MSUD is caused by a deficiency of the branched chain α-ketoacid dehydrogenase complex which requires five cofactors (thiamine, riboflavin, niacin, pantothenic acid and lipoic acid)**
- **Administration of any of the cofactors could theoretically improve this patient's condition**
- **However, only thiamine is used clinically**

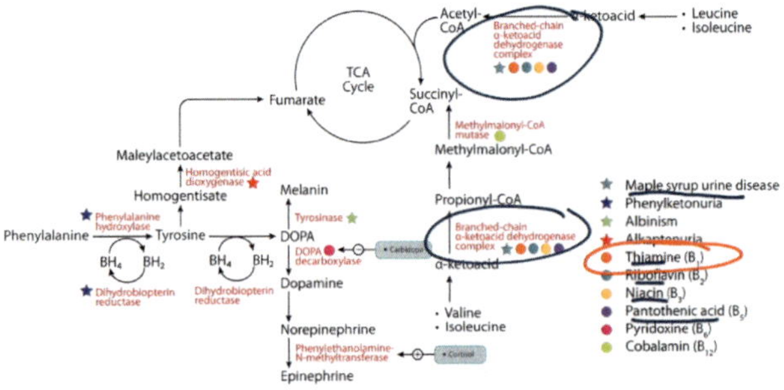

2. A 6-month-old boy is brought to the physician for seizures and developmental delay. His parents state that they adopted him from out of the country and he was brought to the united States a few weeks ago. On exam he has a musty body odor and a fair complexion. An enzyme deficiency is suspected and dietary restriction along with tyrosine supplementation is recommended. However, the parents return two weeks later due to worsening of his condition. Based on this patient's enzymatic deficiency, how would smooth muscle relaxation likely be altered compared to a healthy individual?

- **In classic phenylketonuria treatment includes phenylalanine restriction and dietary supplementation with tyrosine**
- **This treatment was not effective → symptoms are likely due to a dihydrobiopterin reductase deficiency**
- **The conversion of arginine → nitric oxide requires dihydrobiopterin reductase**
- **A deficiency results in ↓ nitric oxide synthesis (normally causes smooth muscle relaxation) → ↓ smooth muscle relaxation**

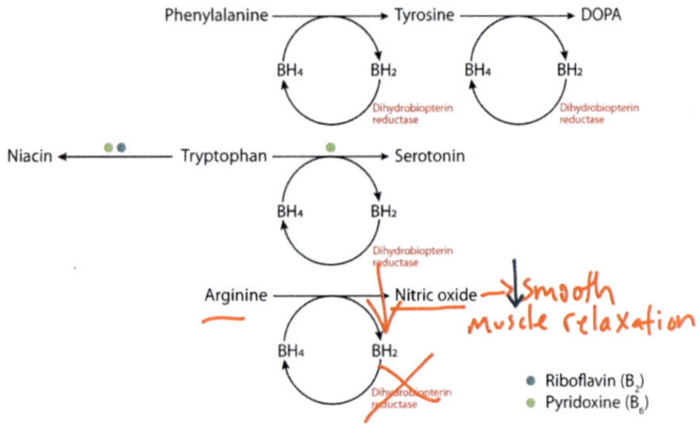

3. A 3-week-old boy is brought to the pediatrician for a follow up visit. As the interview progresses the mother brings up a concern about her boy's diaper appearing black after he urinates. An enzyme deficiency is suspected. What is a likely complication that will occur as this boy gets older?

- **Black urine (black diaper after urinating) → alkaptonuria → deposition of homogentisic acid in joints → arthritis**

Section XIX - Lysosomal Storage Diseases

I. Overview

A. Lysosomes breakdown obsolete components of the cell.

B. Lysosomal storage diseases are caused by an absence of lysosomal enzymes that metabolize sphingolipids.

C. Sphingolipids are associated with nerve tissue.

II. Lysosomal storage diseases (Table 2.5.3)

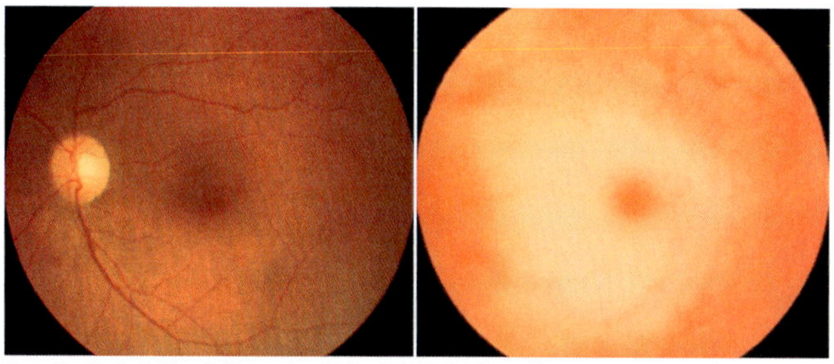

Photo Credit: By Tmhlee (left), Jonathan Trobe, M.D. (right) (https://creativecommons.org)

Left: Normal retina, Right: Cherry-red spot

Disease	Deficient Enzyme	Accumulated Substrate	Findings	Inheritance
Fabry disease "Fa - br - A"	α-galactosidase A	Ceramide trihexoside	- Palm and sole neuropathy - ↓ autonomics (sweat) - Renal and CV failure in adulthood - Angiokeratoma	X-linked recessive
Niemann-Pick disease "No man picks his nose with his sphinger"	Sphingomyelinase	Sphingomyelin	- Weakness - Cherry-red spot - Hepatosplenomegaly - Foam cells	Autosomal recessive
Tay-Sachs disease "Tay-SaX lacks hexosaMinidase"	Hexosaminidase A	GM_2 ganglioside	- Weakness - Cherry-red spot - Lysosomes with onion skin	Autosomal recessive
Gaucher disease "GaUcher"	Glucocerebrosidase	Glucocerebroside	- Bone disease - Lipid-laden macrophages - Pancytopenia	Autosomal recessive
Krabbe disease	Galactocerebrosidase	Galactocerebroside	- Weakness - Vision problems (no cherry-red spot)	Autosomal recessive
Metachromatic leukodystrophy	Arylsulfatase A	Cerebroside sulfate	- Weakness - Dementia - Neuropathy	Autosomal recessive

Table 2.5.3 - Lysosomal storage diseases

REVIEW QUESTIONS

1. A 20-year-old male presents to the physician for recent onset polyuria and polydipsia. Labs are significant for proteinuria and an elevated creatinine. Further investigation reveals a deficiency of an enzyme normally present in lysosomes. What other symptoms would likely accompany the disorder described in this vignette?

- **Polyuria, polydipsia, proteinuria, and an elevated creatinine → renal failure**
- **Fabry disease is the only lysosomal storage disease that results in renal failure**
- **Other symptoms of Fabry disease include palm and sole neuropathy, decreased sweat, cardiovascular failure, and angiokeratomas**

2. A 16-month-old boy is brought to the physician for developmental delay. His parents are a young Ashkenazi Jewish couple who state that he is still unable to walk or crawl. Physical exam reveals hypotonia, hepatosplenomegaly, and a cherry-red spot on fundoscopic exam. A deficiency of what enzyme is most likely the cause of this patient's disease?

- **Weakness, hepatosplenomegaly, and a cherry-red spot → Niemann-Pick disease → deficiency of sphingomyelinase**

Section XIX.1 - Tay-Sachs & Niemann-Pick Disease

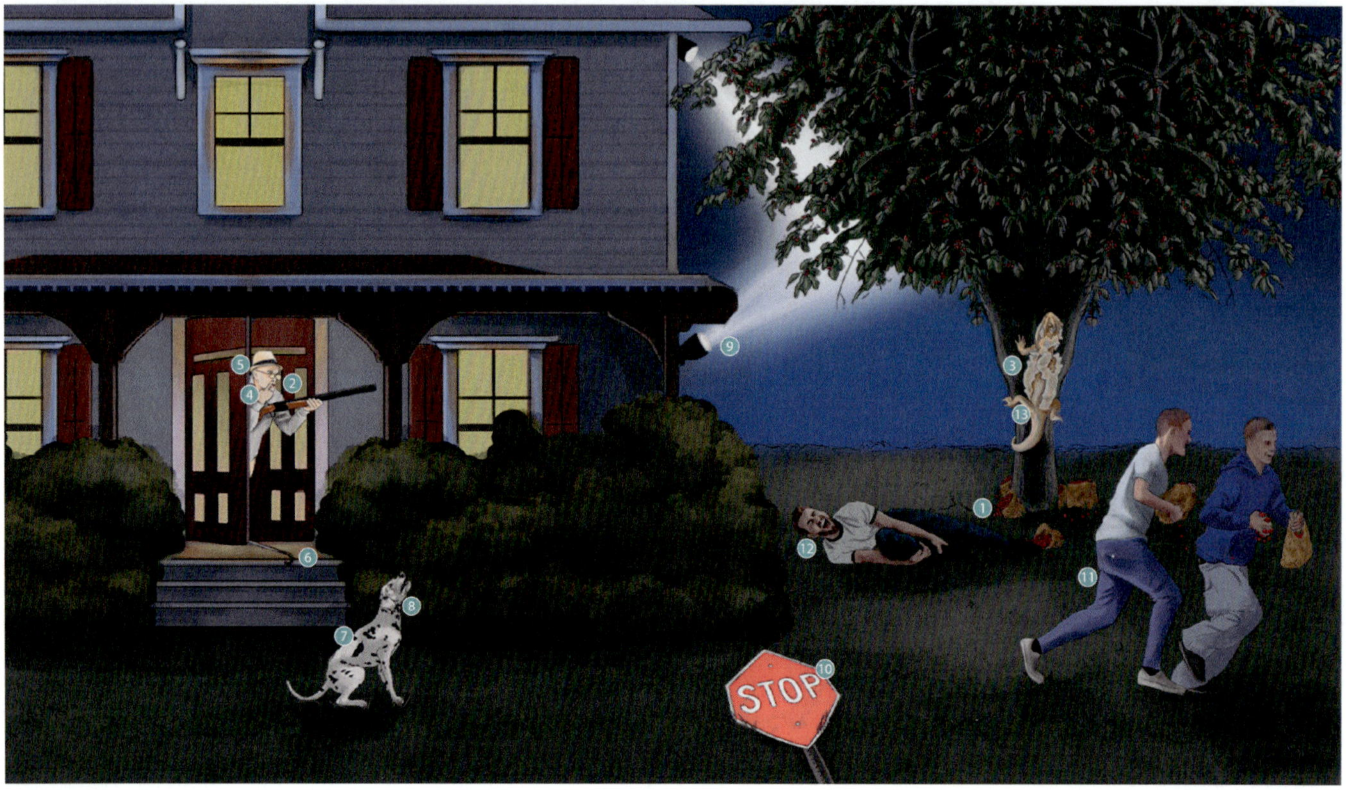

1. ____________________
2. ____________________
3. ____________________
4. ____________________
5. ____________________
6. ____________________
7. ____________________
8. ____________________
9. ____________________
10. ____________________
11. ____________________
12. ____________________
13. ____________________

Section XIX.2 - Fabry Disease

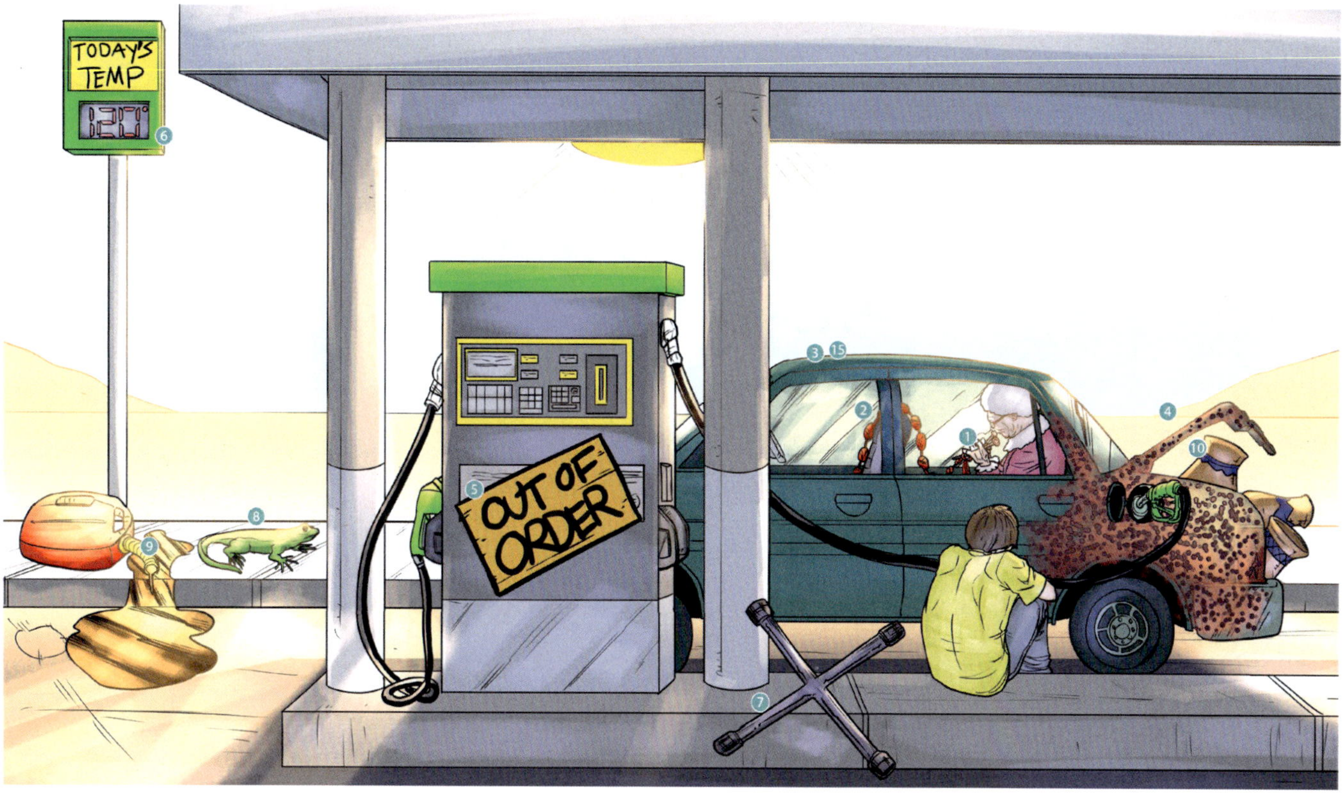

1. ______________________
2. ______________________
3. ______________________
4. ______________________
5. ______________________
6. ______________________
7. ______________________
8. ______________________
9. ______________________
10. ______________________

Section XIX.3 - Metachromatic Leukodystrophy

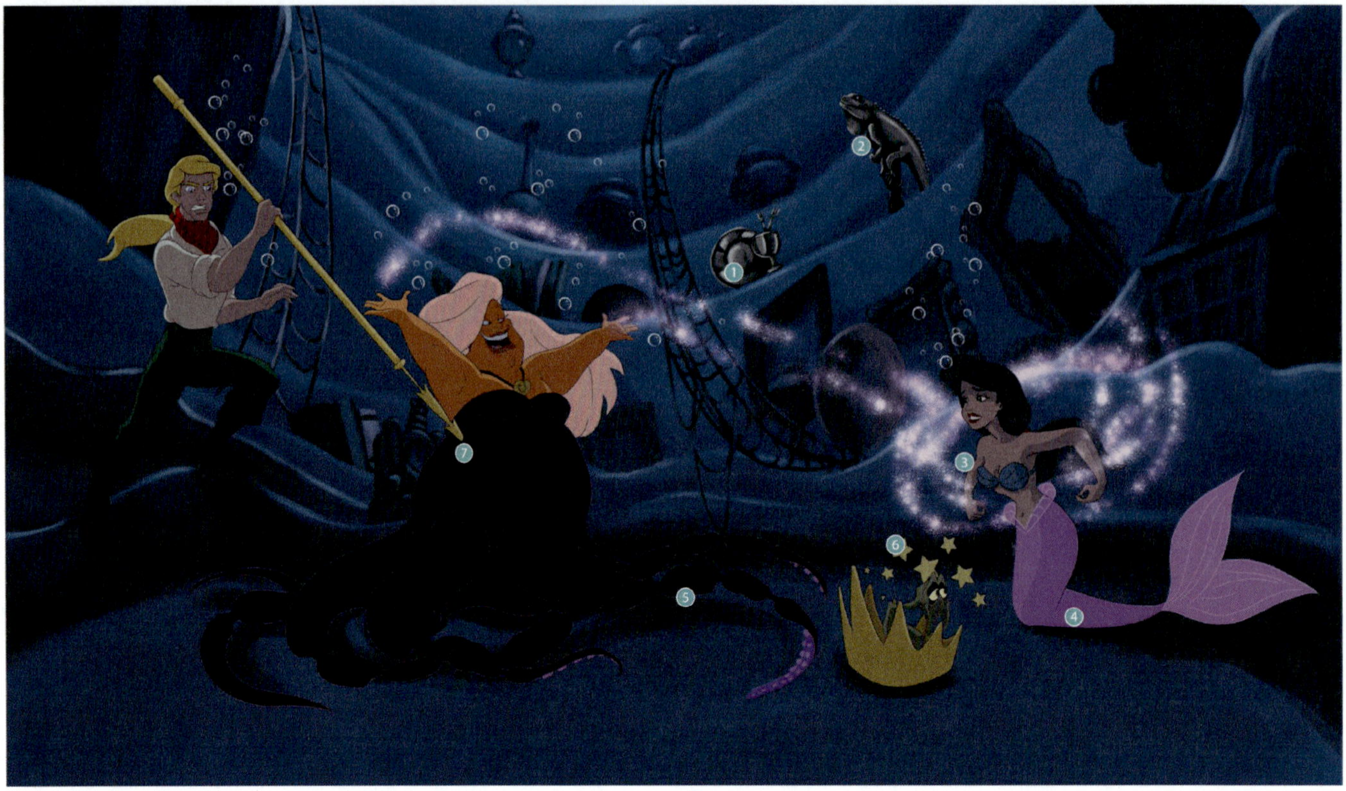

1. ______________________________
2. ______________________________
3. ______________________________
4. ______________________________
5. ______________________________
6. ______________________________
7. ______________________________

Section XIX.4 - Krabbe Disease

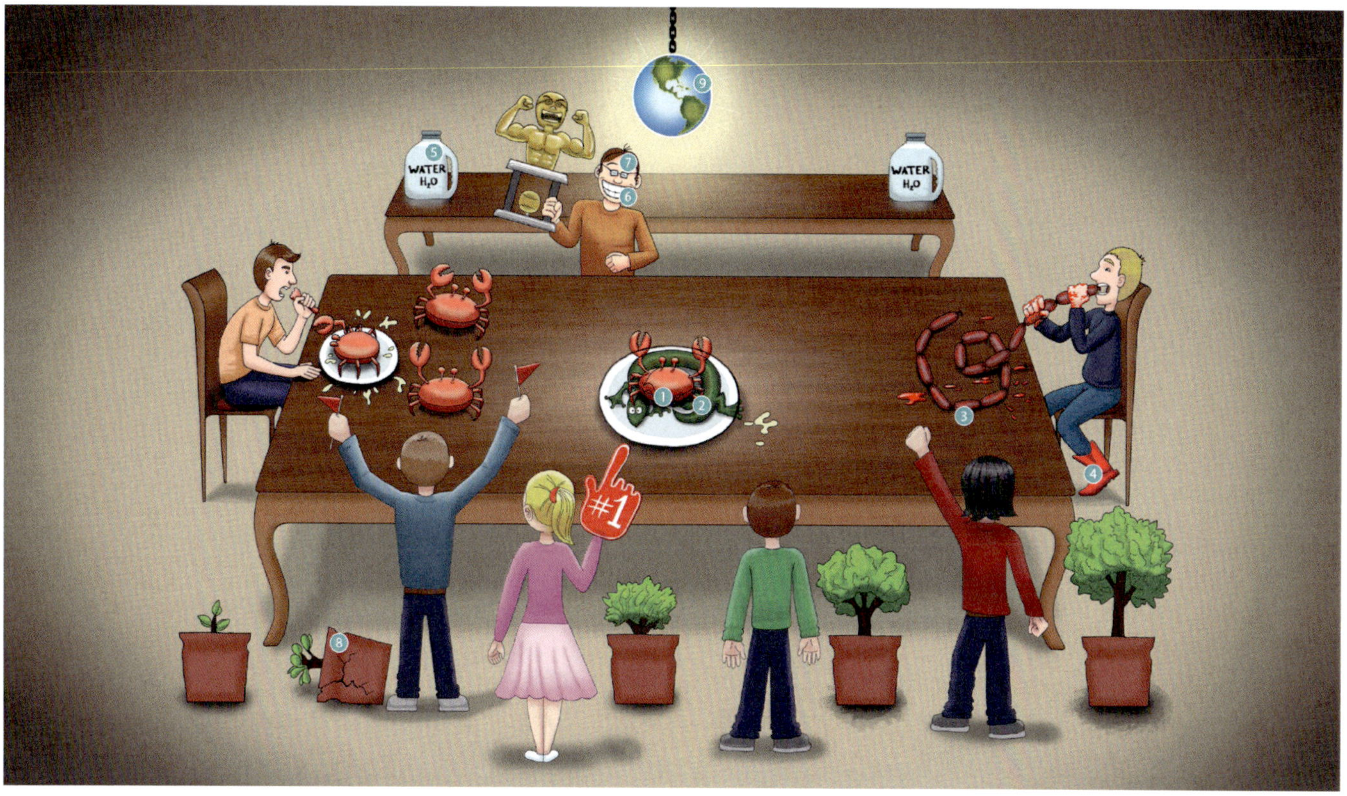

1. ______________________
2. ______________________
3. ______________________
4. ______________________
5. ______________________
6. ______________________
7. ______________________
8. ______________________
9. ______________________

Section XIX.5 - Gaucher Disease

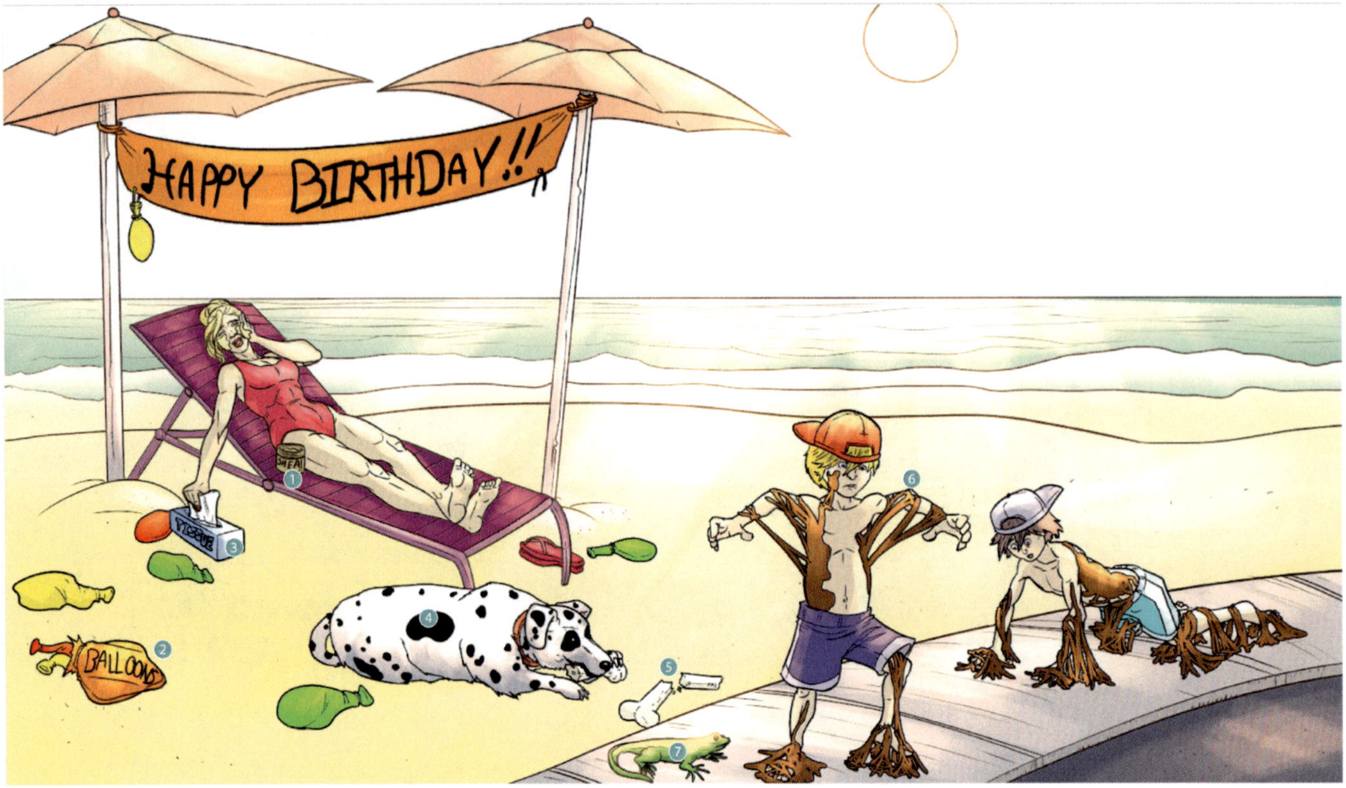

1. ______________________________

2. ______________________________

3. ______________________________

4. ______________________________

5. ______________________________

6. ______________________________

7. ______________________________

Section XIX.6 - Hurler & Hunter Syndrome

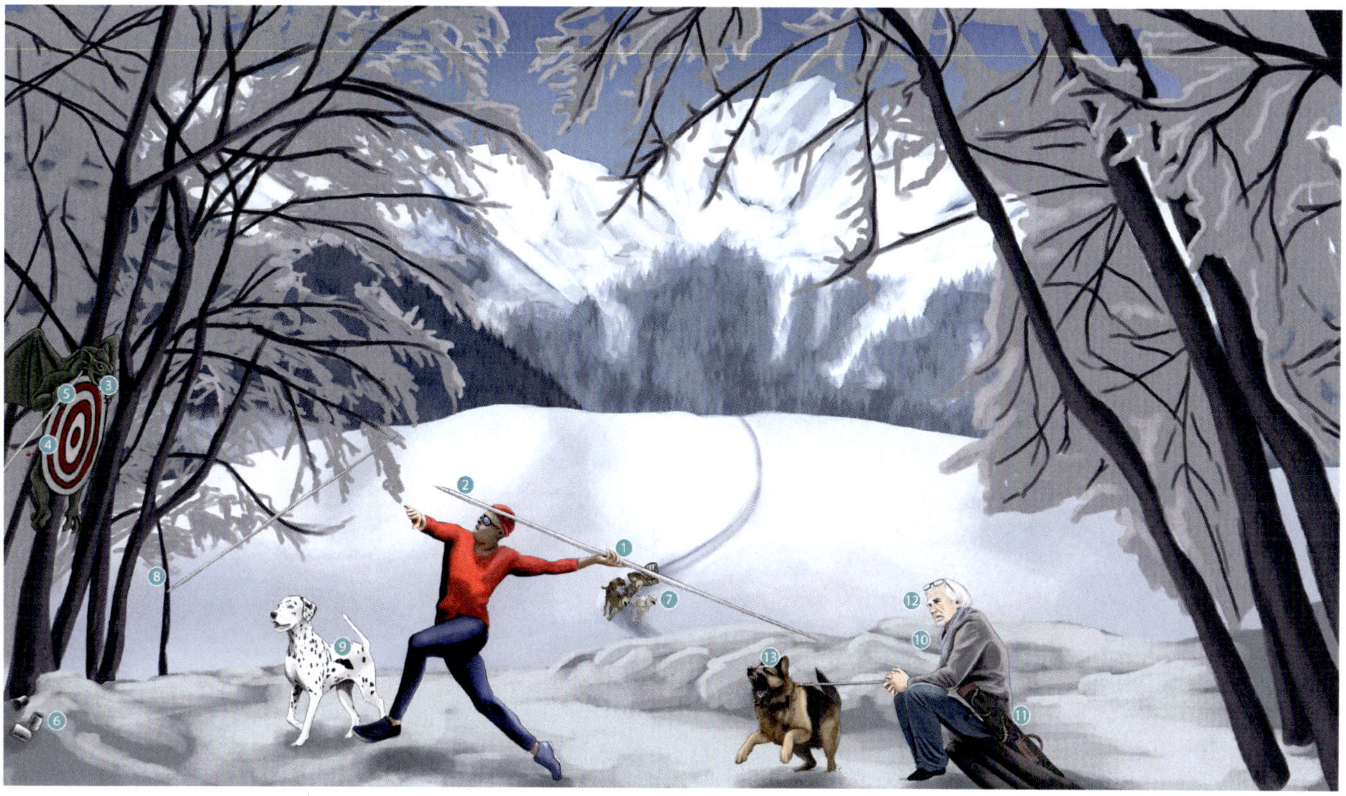

1. ____________________
2. ____________________
3. ____________________
4. ____________________
5. ____________________
6. ____________________
7. ____________________
8. ____________________
9. ____________________
10. ____________________
11. ____________________
12. ____________________
13. ____________________

Section XX - Nutrition

I. Vitamins (Table 2.5.4)

Vitamin	Function	Deficiency	Notes
B_1 (thiamine)	Cofactor for many dehydrogenase enzymes and transketolase	Wernicke-Korsakoff syndrome	• Commonly seen in alcoholism and malnutrition
B_2 (riboflavin)	Cofactor for many dehydrogenase enzymes, necessary for FAD synthesis	Cheilosis and corneal vascularization	
B_3 (niacin)	Cofactor for many dehydrogenase enzymes, necessary for NAD synthesis	Diarrhea, dermatitis, and dementia (excess → facial flushing due to prostaglandin)	• Derived from tryptophan • Hartnup disease
B_5 (pantothenic acid)	Cofactor for many dehydrogenase enzymes	Dermatitis, alopecia, and enteritis	
B_6 (pyridoxine)	Cofactor for transamination reactions, cystathionine synthase, DOPA decarboxylase, serotonin synthesis, niacin synthesis, GABA synthesis, and heme synthesis	Peripheral neuropathy	• Isoniazid induces deficiency
B_7 (biotin)	Cofactor for carboxylase enzymes (i.e. pyruvate carboxylase, acetyl-CoA carboxylase, and propionyl-CoA carboxylase)	Dermatitis, alopecia, and enteritis	• Avidin in egg whites binds biotin
B_9 (folate)	Converted to THF (nucleic acid synthesis, homocysteine, and methylmalonic acid metabolism)	Megaloblastic anemia, ↑ homocysteine, and normal methylmalonic acid levels	• Found in green leafy vegetables
B_{12} (cobalamin)	Cofactor for methionine synthase and methylmalonyl-CoA mutase	Megaloblastic anemia, ↑ homocysteine, ↑ methylmalonic acid levels, and subacute combined degeneration	• Found in animal products
Vitamin C	Collagen synthesis	Swollen gums, petechiae, and poor wound healing	• Found in fruits and vegetables
Vitamin A	Vision and normal differentiation of epithelial cells	Night blindness, dry skin, and keratomalacia (excess → ↑ ICP & dry skin)	• Isotretinoin used to treat cystic acne • All-trans retinoic acid used to treat APL
Vitamin D	Calcium and phosphate regulation	Rickets and osteomalacia (excess → hypercalcemia)	• Formed in sun-exposed epithelium
Vitamin E	Protects RBCs	Anemia and neurological deficits	• MCV is <100
Vitamin K	Clotting	Neonatal hemorrhage	• Produced by colonic bacteria

Table 2.5.4 - Vitamins

II. Hartnup disease

A. Deficiency of neutral amino acid transporters (tryptophan) in the kidneys and small intestine.

B. Tryptophan is a precursor for niacin.

C. ↓ niacin → pellagra (dermatitis, diarrhea, and dementia)

III. Malnutrition

A. Kwashiorkor

1. ↓ protein → ↓ apolipoprotein synthesis → fatty liver → ↓ oncotic pressure → edema

A. Marasmus

B. ↓ calories → tissue and muscle wasting

REVIEW QUESTIONS

1. A 10-year-old boy presents with a three week history of watery diarrhea. He also has been irritable and has had a pruritic rash during this time. Labs are significant for elevated neutral amino acids in the urine. How would the activity of α-ketoglutarate dehydrogenase in this patient likely compare to that of a healthy individual?

- **↑ neutral amino acids in the urine → Hartnup disease → ↓ tryptophan (precursor to niacin) → pellagra (dermatitis, diarrhea, and dementia)**
- **Niacin is a cofactor for α-ketoglutarate dehydrogenase so a deficiency of niacin would result in decreased activity of this enzyme compared to a healthy individual**

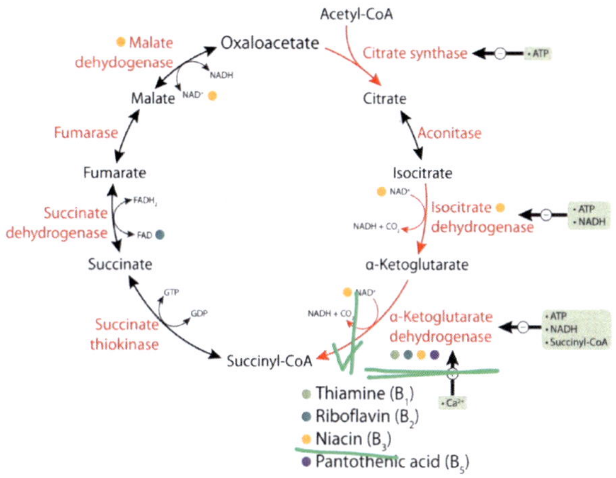

2. A 55-year-old male with a history of heavy alcohol and tobacco use presents to the physician due to a 3-week history of unstable gait, numbness and tingling in the extremities, and generalized weakness. Physical examination reveals ataxia, decreased proprioception, and bilateral weakness. Stool analysis reveals an increased fat concentration. CT of the abdomen shows a mass concerning for malignancy. Which of the following is most likely deficient in this patient?

   A) Vitamin B_6 (pyridoxine)
   B) Vitamin E
   C) Vitamin B_{12} (cobalamin)
   D) Vitamin B_1 (thiamine)
   E) Vitamin B_9 (folate)
   F) Vitamin A

- **Increased fat concentration in the stool, an abdominal mass, and a history of alcohol and tobacco use → pancreatic malignancy → fat malabsorption**
- **Neurological deficits → vitamin E deficiency**

Section XX.1 - Thiamine

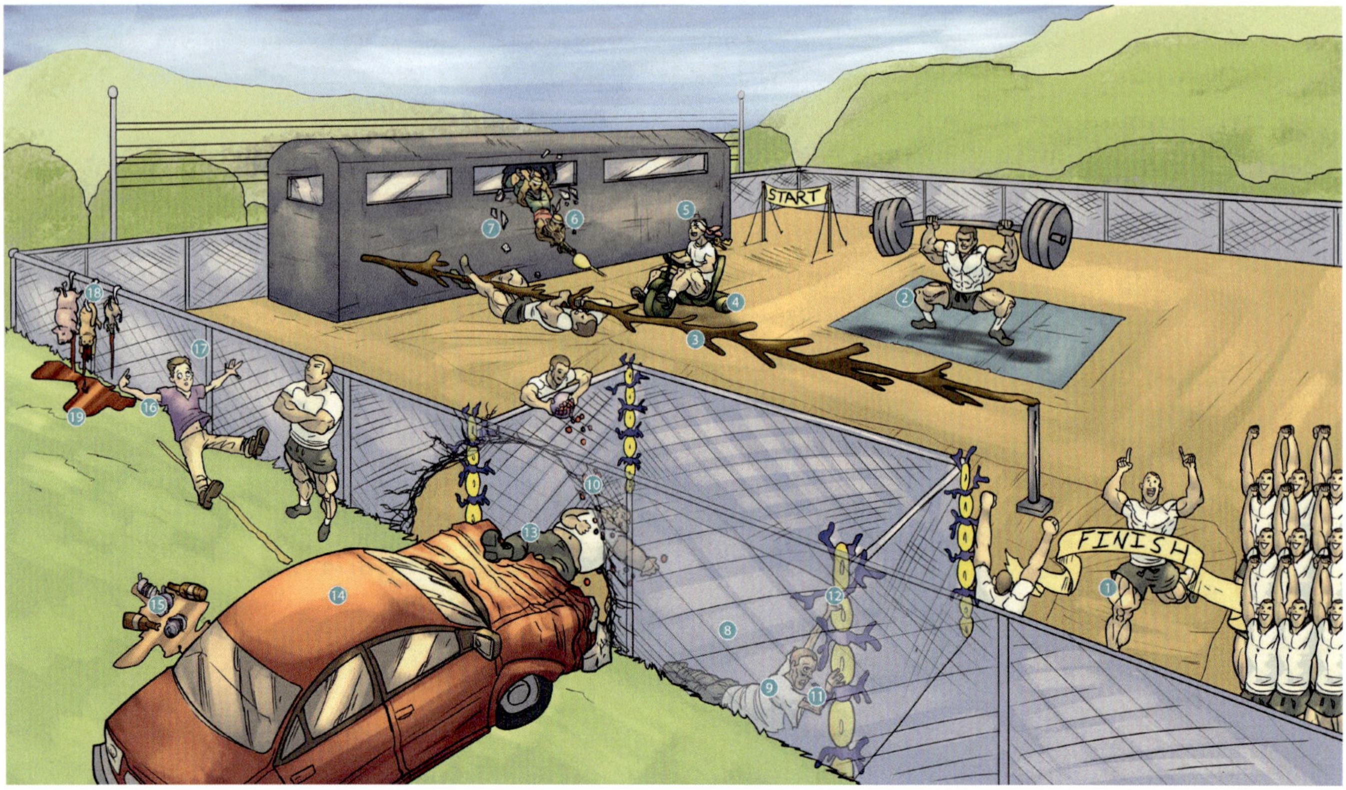

1. ______________________
2. ______________________
3. ______________________
4. ______________________
5. ______________________
6. ______________________
7. ______________________
8. ______________________
9. ______________________
10. ______________________
11. ______________________
12. ______________________
13. ______________________
14. ______________________
15. ______________________
16. ______________________
17. ______________________
18. ______________________
19. ______________________

Section XX.2 - Riboflavin (B2)

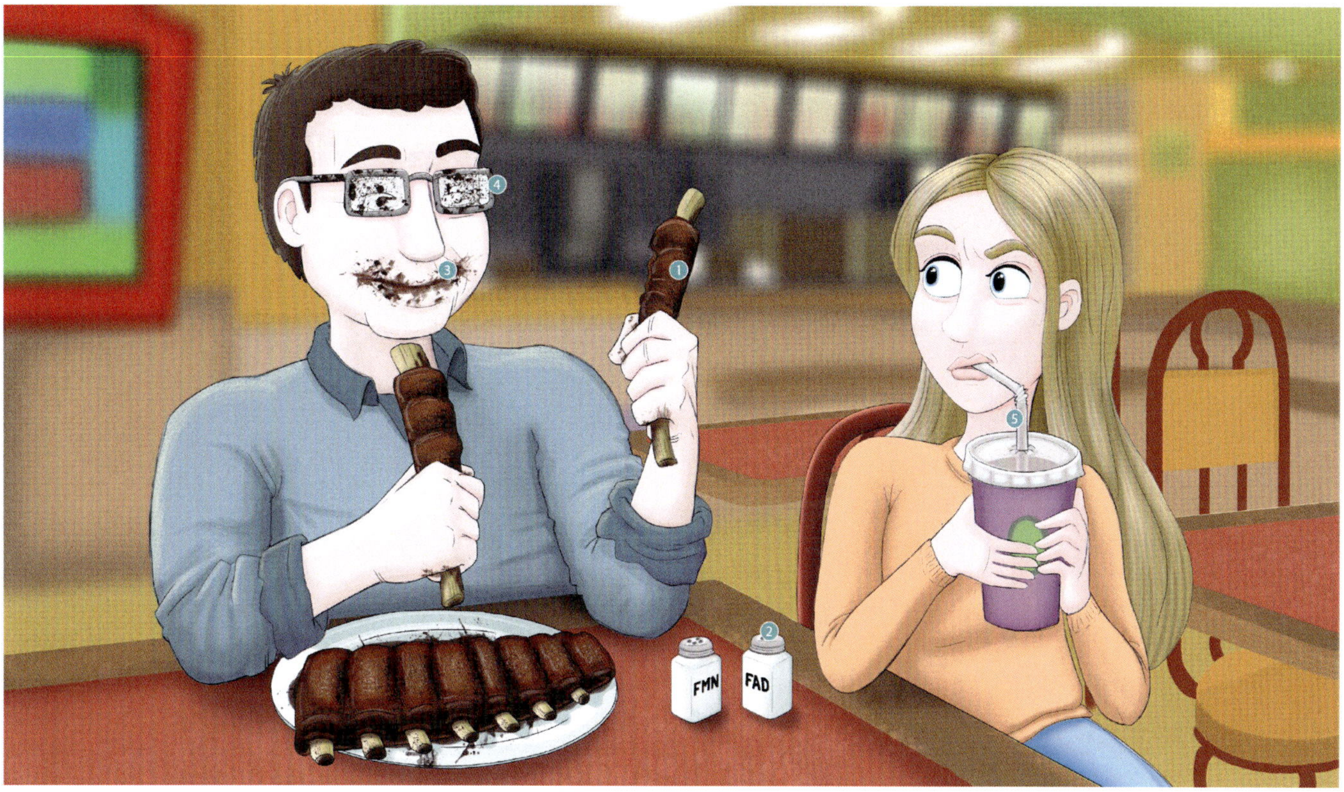

1. ______________________________
2. ______________________________
3. ______________________________
4. ______________________________
5. ______________________________

Section XX.3 - Niacin (B3)

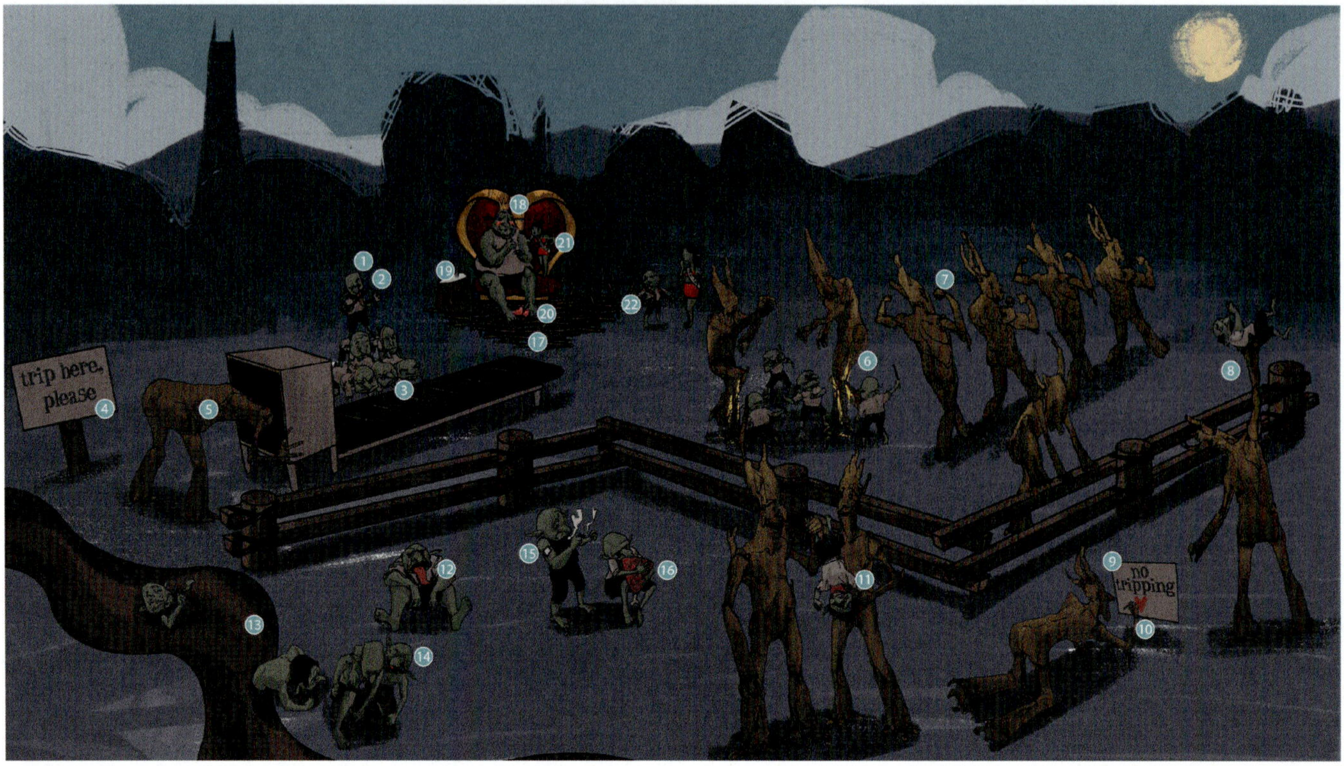

1. ______________________

2. ______________________

3. ______________________

4. ______________________

5. ______________________

6. ______________________

7. ______________________

8. ______________________

9. ______________________

10. ______________________

11. ______________________

12. ______________________

13. ______________________

14. ______________________

15. ______________________

16. ______________________

17. ______________________

18. ______________________

19. ______________________

20. ______________________

21. ______________________

22. ______________________

Section XX.4 - Pantothenic Acid (B5)

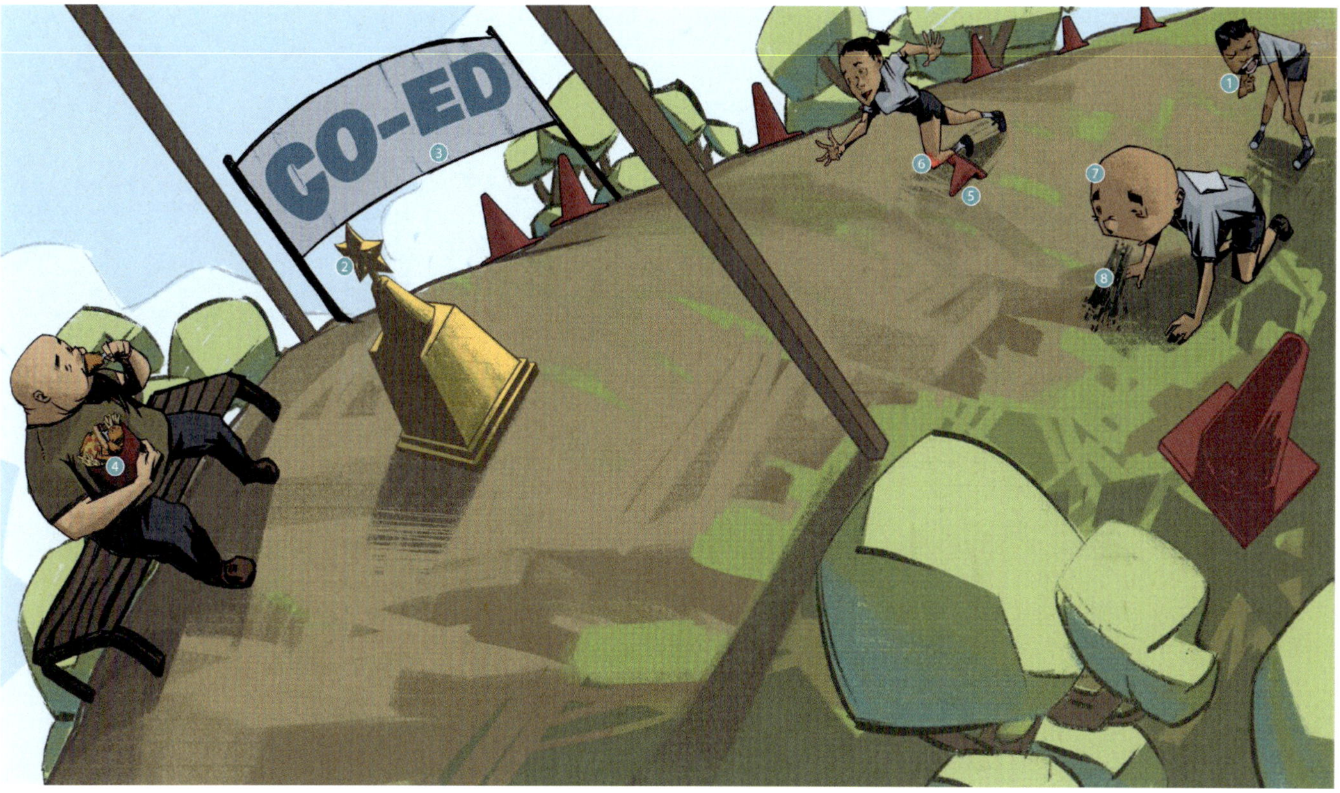

1. ____________________
2. ____________________
3. ____________________
4. ____________________
5. ____________________
6. ____________________
7. ____________________
8. ____________________

Section XX.5 - Pyridoxine (B6)

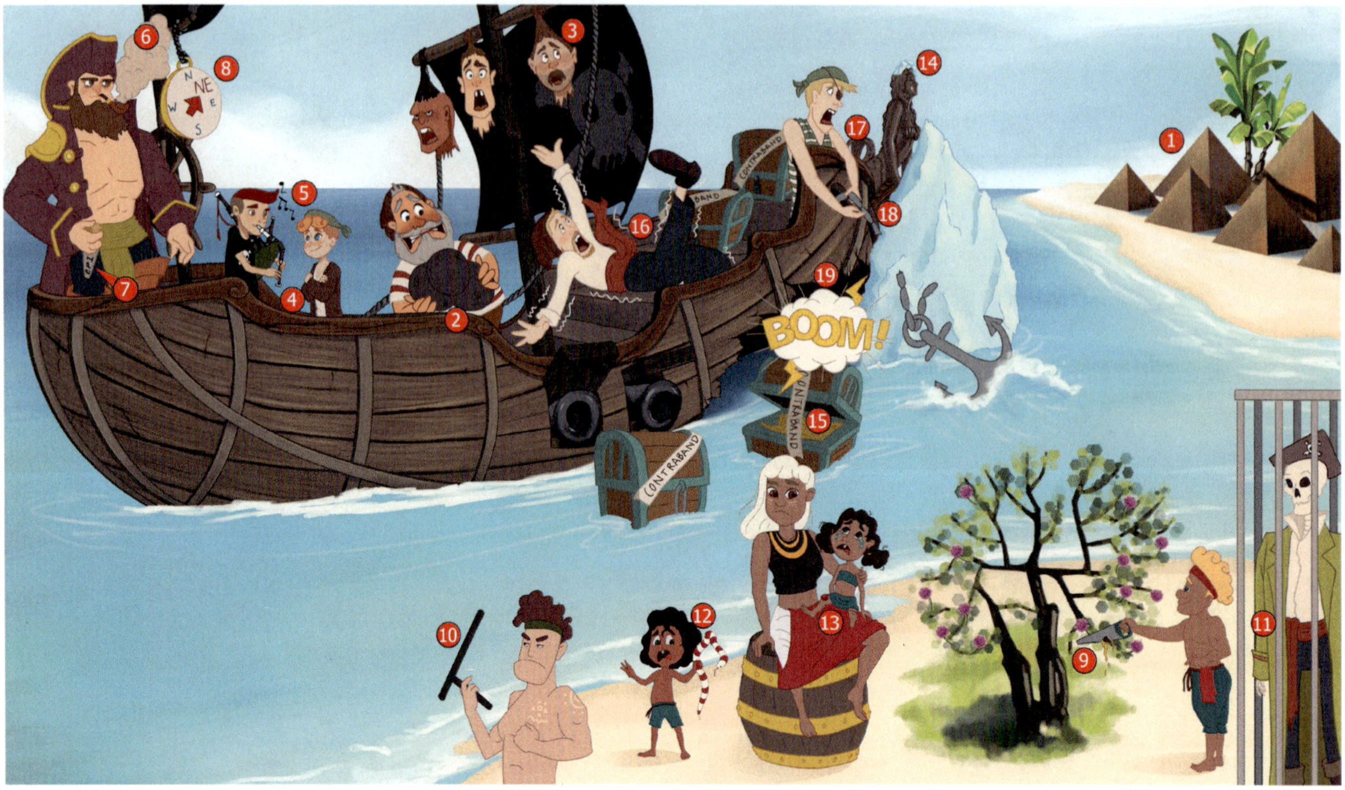

1. Six pyramids: Pyridoxine (Vitamin B_6)

2. Pirate carrying ammo: Pyridoxine is a cofactor used for transamination (e.g. AST and ALT)

3. Decapitated heads: Pyridoxine is a cofactor for decarboxylation reactions

4. Gabe waiting: Pyridoxine is a cofactor for the production of GABA

5. Friends sharing tunes: Pyridoxine is a cofactor in the production of Serotonin

6. Muscular captian smoking dope: Pyridoxine is a cofactor in the production of Dopamine

7.Captian's Epipen: Pyridoxine is a cofactor for the production of Epinephrine

8. Compass pointing northeast on a pirate ship full of pirates ready for a fight: Pyridoxine is a cofactor in the production of Norepinephrine

9. Islander sawing off the most distal branch of the tree: Pyridoxine is a cofactor for the production of glycogen phosphorylase

10. Nightstick: Pyridoxine is a cofactor for Niacin

11. Skeleton with a red scarf in an iron cage: Pyridoxine is a cofactor for the production of heme

12. Hissing snake: Pyridoxine is a cofactor in the production of Histamine

13. Little girl's cyst on her thigh and her glute on her mother's thigh: Pyridoxine is a cofactor in the production of Cystathionine and Glutathione

14. Ice on mermaid's head: Isoniazid can induce functional pyridoxine deficiency

15. Contraband: Contraceptives can induce pyridoxine deficiency

16. Seizing pirate: Pyriodoxine deficiency can cause seizures

17. Irritated pirate: Pyridoxine deficiency can cuase irritability

18. Sausage-link anchor geting detached from the ship: Pyridoxine deficiency can cause peripheral neuropathy

19. Side blast in the pirate ship: Pyridoxine deficiency can cuase sideroblastic anemia

Section XX.6 - Biotin (B7)

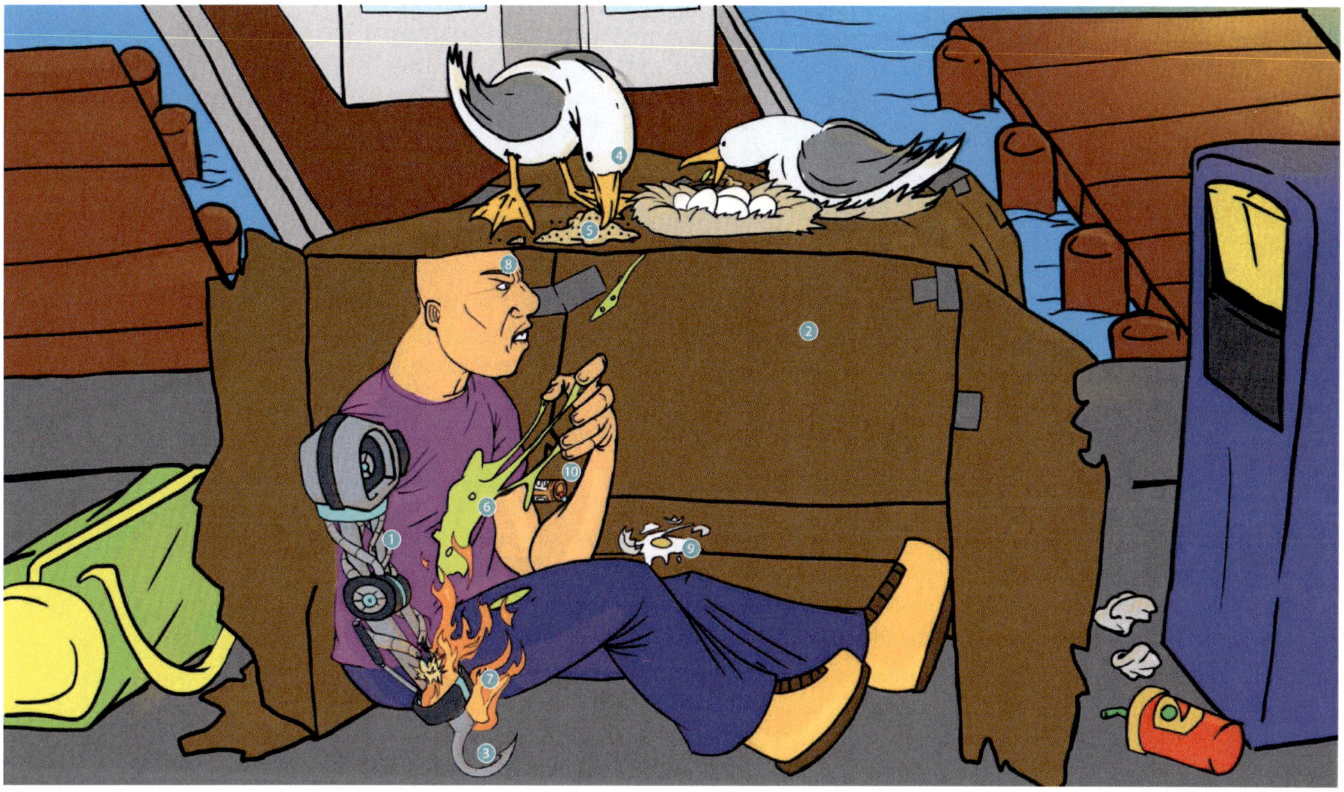

1. ______________________
2. ______________________
3. ______________________
4. ______________________
5. ______________________
6. ______________________
7. ______________________
8. ______________________
9. ______________________
10. ______________________

Section XX.7 - Folate (B9)

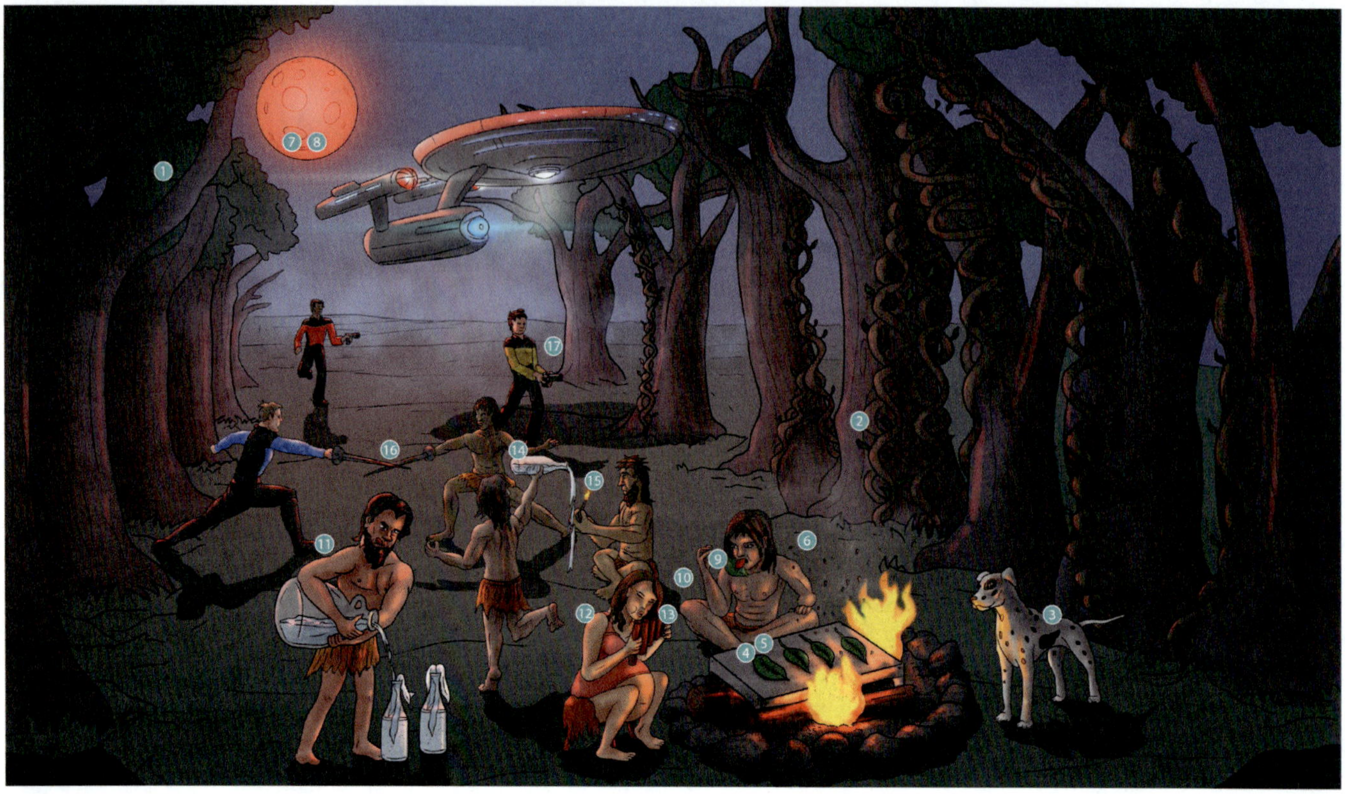

1. ______________________
2. ______________________
3. ______________________
4. ______________________
5. ______________________
6. ______________________
7. ______________________
8. ______________________
9. ______________________
10. ______________________
11. ______________________
12. ______________________
13. ______________________
14. ______________________
15. ______________________
16. ______________________
17. ______________________

Section XX.8 - Cobalamin (B12)

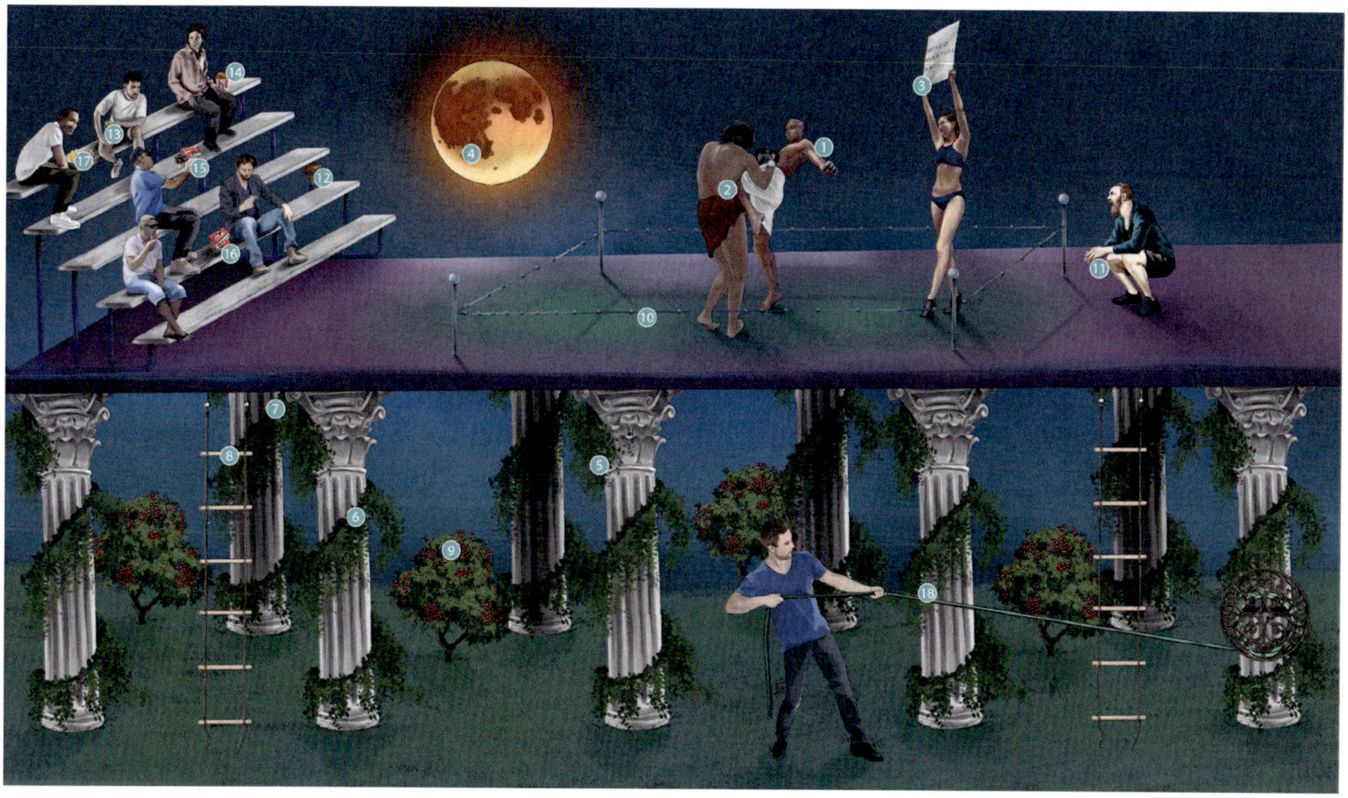

1. __________
2. __________
3. __________
4. __________
5. __________
6. __________
7. __________
8. __________
9. __________
10. __________
11. __________
12. __________
13. __________
14. __________
15. __________
16. __________
17. __________
18. __________

Section XX.9 - Vitamin C

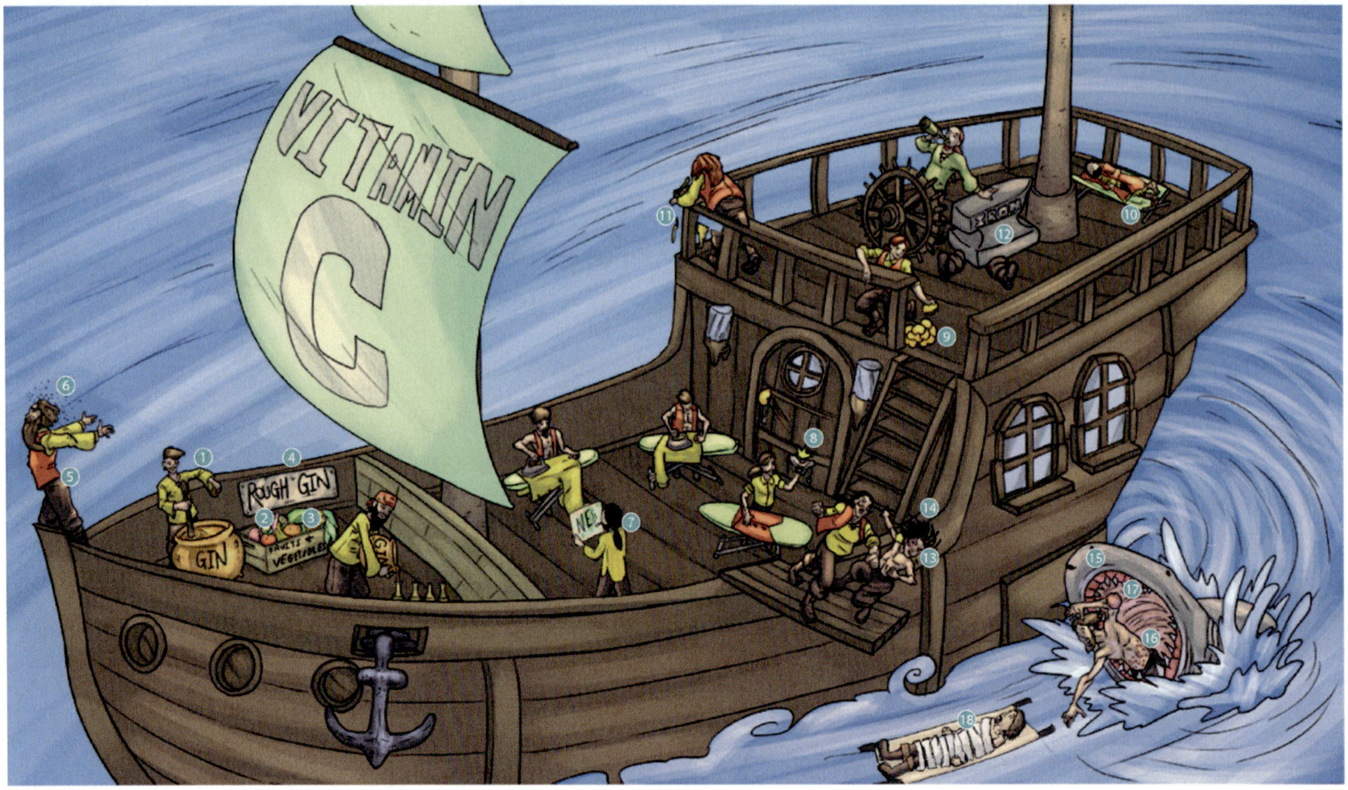

1. ____________________
2. ____________________
3. ____________________
4. ____________________
5. ____________________
6. ____________________
7. ____________________
8. ____________________
9. ____________________
10. ____________________
11. ____________________
12. ____________________
13. ____________________
14. ____________________
15. ____________________
16. ____________________
17. ____________________
18. ____________________

Section XX.10 - Vitamin A

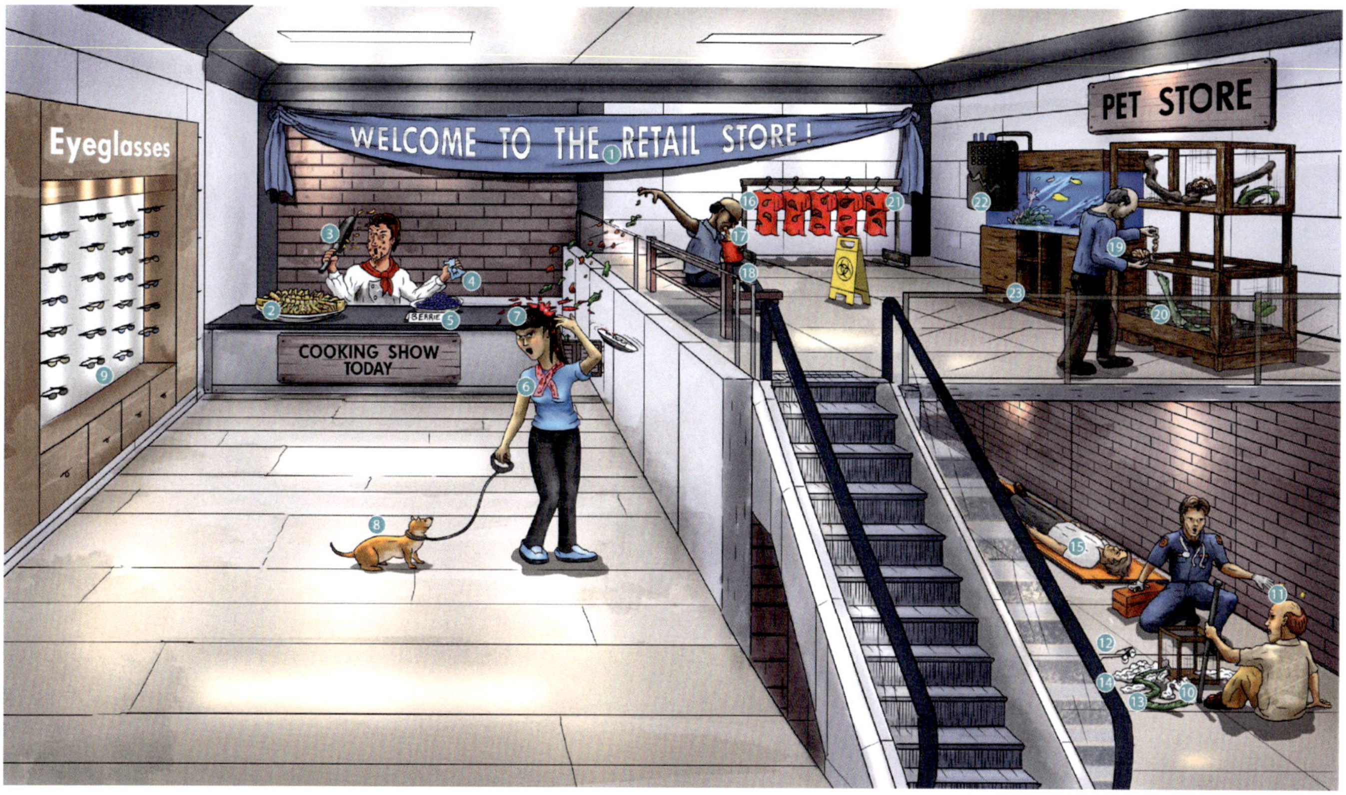

1. ______________________
2. ______________________
3. ______________________
4. ______________________
5. ______________________
6. ______________________
7. ______________________
8. ______________________
9. ______________________
10. ______________________
11. ______________________
12. ______________________
13. ______________________
14. ______________________
15. ______________________
16. ______________________
17. ______________________
18. ______________________
19. ______________________
20. ______________________
21. ______________________
22. ______________________
23. ______________________

Section XX.11 - Vitamin D

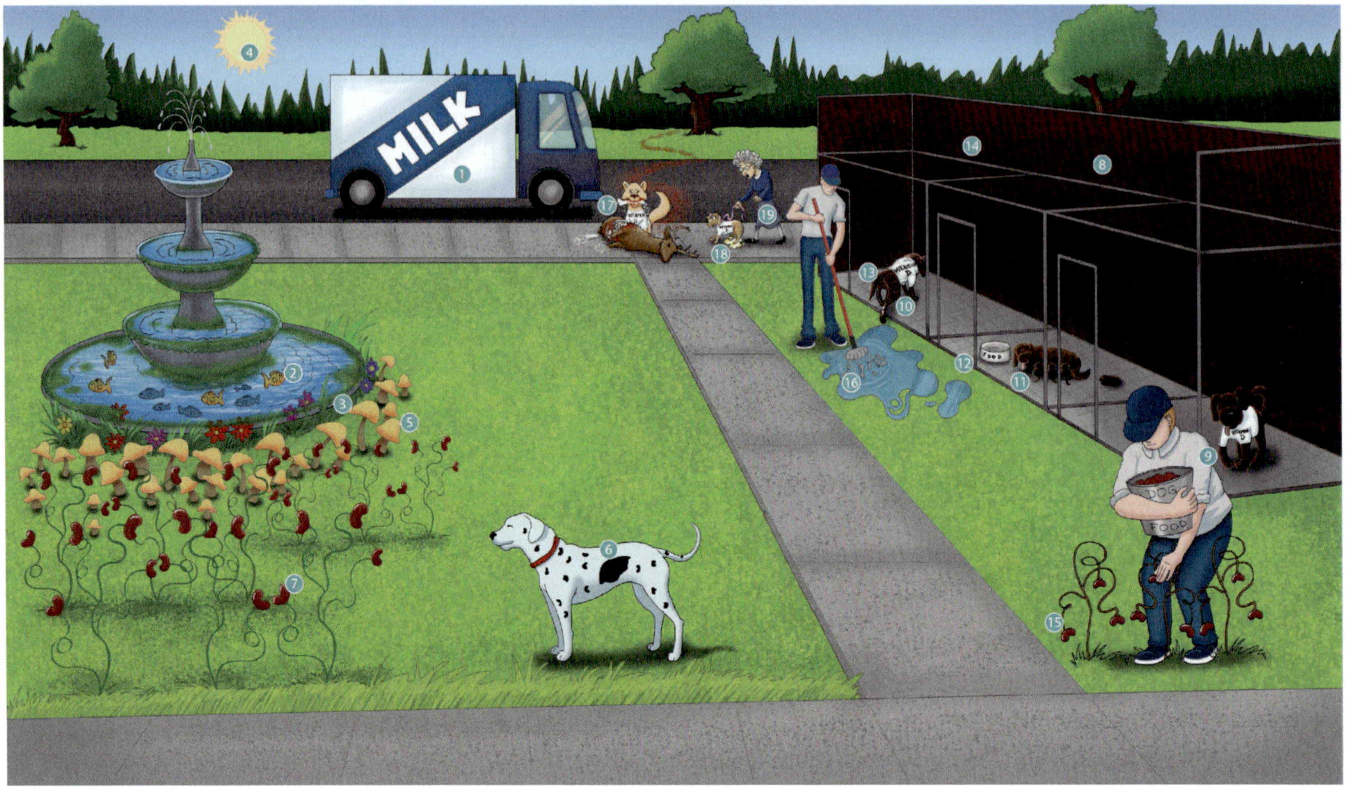

1. ______________________

2. ______________________

3. ______________________

4. ______________________

5. ______________________

6. ______________________

7. ______________________

8. ______________________

9. ______________________

10. ______________________

11. ______________________

12. ______________________

13. ______________________

14. ______________________

15. ______________________

16. ______________________

17. ______________________

18. ______________________

19. ______________________

Section XX.12 - Vitamin E

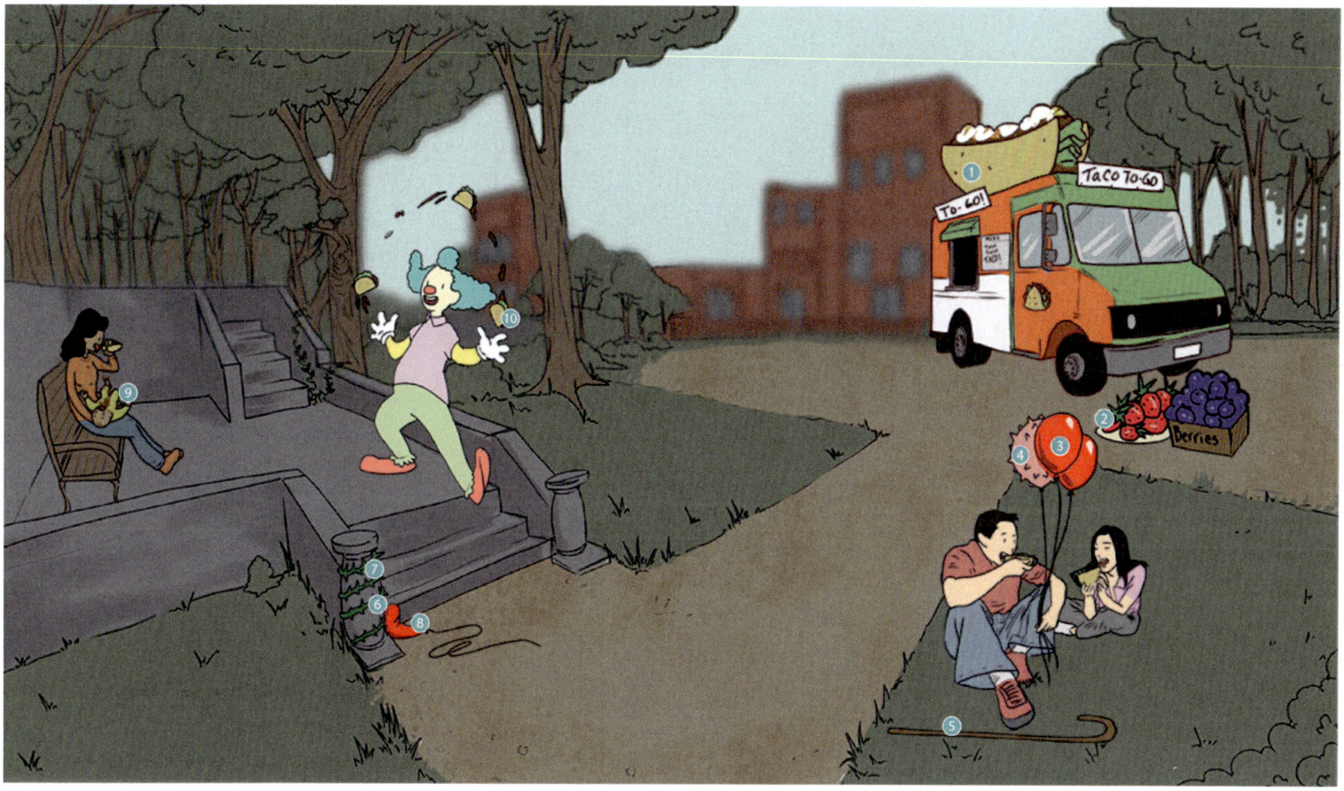

1. ______________________
2. ______________________
3. ______________________
4. ______________________
5. ______________________
6. ______________________
7. ______________________
8. ______________________
9. ______________________
10. ______________________

Section XX.13 - Vitamin K

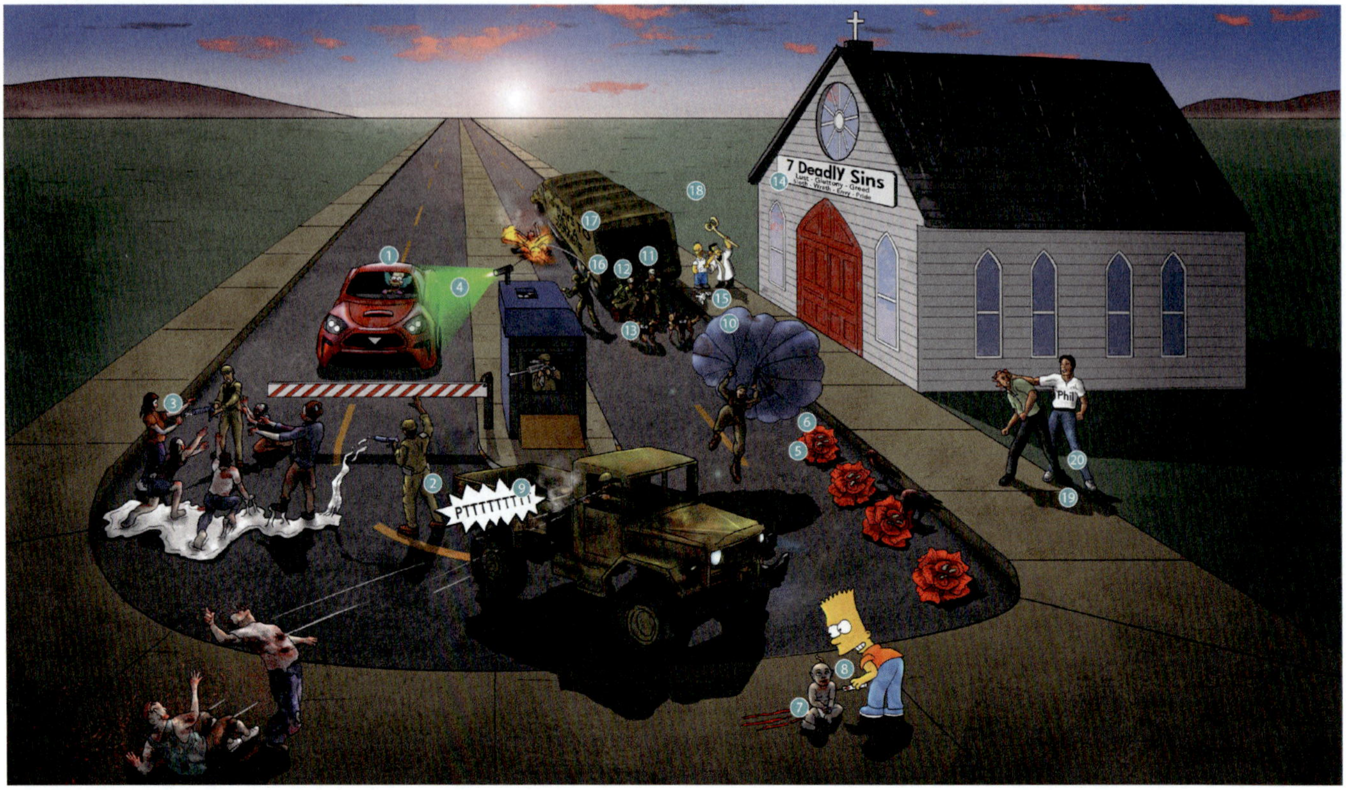

1. ______________________________
2. ______________________________
3. ______________________________
4. ______________________________
5. ______________________________
6. ______________________________
7. ______________________________
8. ______________________________
9. ______________________________
10. ______________________________
11. ______________________________
12. ______________________________
13. ______________________________
14. ______________________________
15. ______________________________
16. ______________________________
17. ______________________________
18. ______________________________
19. ______________________________
20. ______________________________

Section XX.14 - Zinc

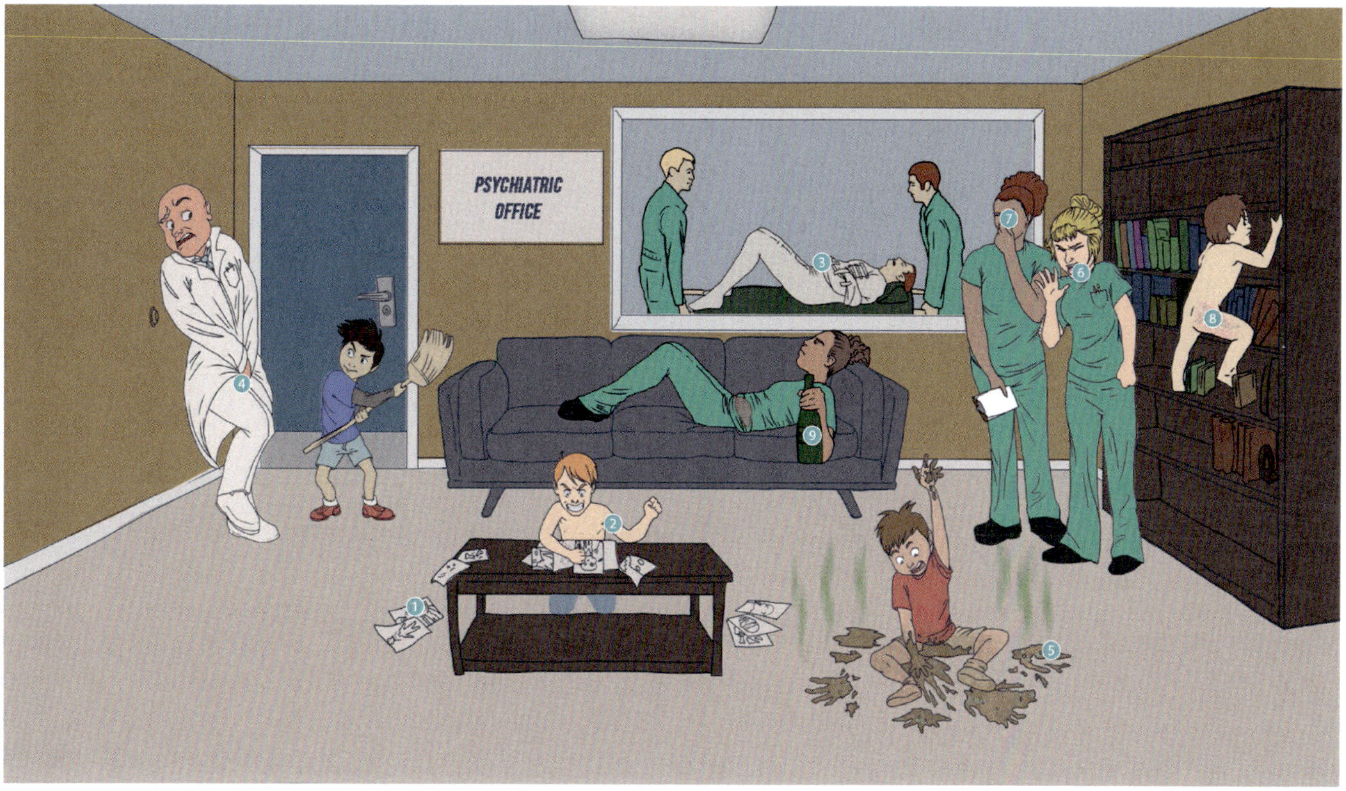

1. ______________________________
2. ______________________________
3. ______________________________
4. ______________________________
5. ______________________________
6. ______________________________
7. ______________________________
8. ______________________________
9. ______________________________

TABLES & FIGURES

INDEX

Symbols

A

B

C

D

E

F

G

O

P

R

S

T

U

V

W

X

Made in United States
Orlando, FL
04 November 2026

90200385R00083